APPETITES

Geneen Roth

·

APPETITES

·

ON THE SEARCH
FOR TRUE
NOURISHMENT

℗

A PLUME BOOK

PLUME
Published by the Penguin Group
Penguin Putnam Inc., 375 Hudson Street, New York, New York 10014, U.S.A.
Penguin Books Ltd, 27 Wrights Lane, London W8 5TZ, England
Penguin Books Australia Ltd, Ringwood, Victoria, Australia
Penguin Books Canada Ltd, 10 Alcorn Avenue, Toronto, Ontario,
Canada M4V 3B2
Penguin Books (N.Z.) Ltd, 182–190 Wairau Road, Auckland 10, New Zealand

Penguin Books Ltd, Registered Offices: Harmondsworth, Middlesex, England

Published by Plume, a member of Penguin Putnam Inc.
Previously published in a Dutton edition.

First Plume Printing, April 1997
20 19 18 17 16 15 14 13 12 11

Grateful acknowledgment is made for permission to reprint the following texts:
"Housing Storage" from *The Dangerous World* by Naomi Replansky (Another Chicago
Press, 1994). © Naomi Replansky. By permission of the author.
Prayers from *Kehilla Community Synagogue Prayerbook*. By permission of Michael Lerner
and the Kehilla Community Synagogue.
Prayers from *Kolaynu Yom Kippur Prayerbook*. By permission of Kolaynu.

(P) REGISTERED TRADEMARK—MARCA REGISTRADA

The Library of Congress has catalogued the Dutton edition as follows:
Roth, Geneen.
Appetites : on the search for true nourishment / Geneen Roth.
p. cm.
ISBN 0-525-94076-6 (hc.)
0-452-27679-9 (pbk.)
1. Women—Mental health. 2. Self-esteem in women. 3. Self-realization.
4. Self-acceptance. 5. Self-perception in women.
6. Leaness—Psychological aspects. I. Title.
RC451.4.W6R68   1996
158'.1'082—dc20   96-10801
CIP

Printed in the United States of America
Original hardcover design by Eve L. Kirch

To Matt, again
and again.

Housing Shortage
NAOMI REPLANSKY

I tried to live small.
I took a narrow bed.
I held my elbows to my sides.
I tried to step carefully
And to think softly
And to breathe shallowly
In my portion of air
And to disturb no one.

Yet see how I spread out and I cannot help it.
I take to myself more and more, and I take nothing
That I do not need, but my needs grow like weeds,
All over and invading; I clutter this place
With all the apparatus of living
You stumble over it daily.

And then my lungs take their fill.
And then you gasp for air.

Excuse me for living,
But, since I am living,
Given inches, I take yards,
Taking yards, dream of miles,
And a landscape, unbounded
And vast in abandon.

You too dreaming the same.

Contents

Prologue:
The Places We Search

When I was eleven years old, I planned the rest of my life. I was going to marry Richard Chamberlain and dress in gowns that glimmered like mermaids' tails. I was going to eat Barriccini's chocolate any time I wanted and have three children: two girls named Elizabeth and Samantha, and a boy named Michael. My legs would be long, my hair would be thick, and my stomach would be flat. Most of all, I would be very, very famous. More famous than anyone, ever.

As I entered the teenage years, I told myself that my task was to endure my life-as-it-was until it metamorphosed into my life-to-be. To put up with smarmy boys and an array of degrading circumstances because sometime in the future I was certain to lead a golden life.

Years passed. My unlived life, like a river that ran parallel to my daily life, continued its course through my mind. Richard Chamberlain became Omar Sharif, who became Harrison Ford; Samantha and Elizabeth were replaced by Jennifer and Rebecca, who were replaced by the conviction that having children was a thorn in the side of feminism. Every ingredient of my life-to-be changed constantly—where I lived, how I dressed, what I did with my time—except the hunger to be seen, the longing to be recognized for something I didn't yet recognize in myself.

Being exaltingly thin was, of course, the foundation for the visibility, the man, the adornments of this life-to-be; it was the prerequisite that made the rest of the dream possible. And since no matter how thin I got, I was frightened that I could wake up tomorrow and be fat again, the rest of the dream was forever ten or twenty pounds away.

I was twenty-eight when I decided I would never diet again. After the initial binges on raw chocolate chip cookies, pumpkin ice cream and chunks of bittersweet chocolate, I started eating things that other people recognized as food. Broccoli, pasta, roast chicken, lentil soup. I got thin enough—and stayed thin.

After that there were two small matters to deal with before the rivers of my two lives could converge: being seen and falling in love.

At thirty-five, I met a man whom I recognized almost instantly as my life's partner. Five years later, I married Matt, and although he is not a movie star, he is often mistaken for one. If you can call Richard Simmons a movie star.

And while I never achieved the clicking-flashbulbs kind of fame, people often stop me in the grocery store because they recognize me from my book covers. They also stop me in airports, elevators, and almost every time my hair is dirty and my clothes are covered with white cat fur.

In one way or another I got what I wanted—the body, the recognition, the man. Still, I felt empty and then crazy for feeling empty. I felt like an ungrateful wretch, a needy child for whom nothing is ever enough. I also felt betrayed: I'd followed all the rules, done what I'd been told, and *something* was supposed to happen. I was supposed to have a clear, solid sense of myself as worthy; I was supposed to feel full, radiant. Instead I found myself wildly alternating between believing I needed more (of everything—love, visibility, things, pleasure, thinness, solitude) to feel satisfied, and feeling as if I had built my life on lies. I felt brittle and exhausted. I became ill with an array of mysterious symptoms: chronic diarrhea, constant flus, high fevers. I spent years in and out of doctors' offices as my body became weaker and weaker. Three of my friends, a well-known writer, an English professor, and a nurse-midwife, were also sick, one of them with lupus, another with recurring pneumonia, and the third with chronic fatigue syndrome. The friends who weren't ill were nonetheless weary and disillusioned from trying to keep up with childhood dreams and cultural imperatives of who they were supposed to be. Their lives were crammed with work, child care, exercise, self-improvement classes, political organizing, but they were left with feelings reminiscent of a binge: full but not satisfied. Full but still hungry. Everyone spoke wistfully about the days when we hadn't needed appointment books to schedule two-hour dinners three weeks in advance.

The doctors' offices were filled with women. Mothers, students, social workers, insurance company executives. Like me, they felt exhausted and deficient, and like me, they were flocking to the doctor of the moment to be healed. I met Kaz Covington one morning when the doctor was an hour and a half late and we'd finished all the *People* magazines in his office. After we exchanged the ritual litany of ailments, we exchanged life stories. Kaz was an assistant district attorney, married to a man she loved and respected, and the mother of two young sons. Her life had worked like a well-oiled machine, each minute accounted for, until she got sick and couldn't get out of bed for two months. "My biggest fear is that I'm going to die without having gotten to the heart of my life or done the one thing that has the most meaning," she said. "The thing is, I was going so fast and accomplishing so much, I never had time to figure out what it was.

"I've always been the good girl and done everything I was supposed to, but now that I've done those things, they don't feel like they were supposed to feel. I love my kids—I do—I love my husband, but I feel used up."

The letters I received from women who'd read my books, thousands of letters each year, echoed the same themes. "What's next?" they asked. "We did what you told us to do—ate when we were hungry, stopped when we were full. We lost weight, but our dieting friends don't like us when we're thin, and we got those promotions at work, but something is still missing. And having children doesn't fill the holes in our chests. Now that we don't want to turn to food, where do we turn? What do we do with the emptiness?"

A woman from Wichita, Kansas, wrote, "I feel as if I've been living in a prison, and everything I've done in my life has been an attempt to furnish the cell with chintz and overstuffed chairs. It never occurred to me that I could actually break out of the narrow, self-confined rules I set for myself or that I could find meaning in places besides the shape of my body or success at work. The sad truth is I don't know where to look."

Neither did I.

Appetites is the story of friends and women with whom I've worked as they questioned the meaning of success, thinness, friendship, and fulfillment. It is also a personal story of my attempts to grapple with physical and emotional pain, and to further understand my beliefs about childhood dreams, deprivation, beauty, safety, and joy.

Why, I asked myself, is an embarrassment of riches embarrassing? Why do most women feel they will lose friends if they lose weight? Why do we feel that we have to have small bodies to have big lives? What feels good about feeling bad? And where do we turn for nourishment when it's not in the places we thought it would be?

Most of us, if being truthful, would say that we are disappointed in life, even if (some of) our dreams have come true. In my friend Natalie's words, we thought we would try hard, get to the finish line, and "a big victory" would be waiting for us. Trying hard was supposed to bring long-lasting happiness, and long-lasting happiness was supposed to be found in best friends and lovers, in work and thin bodies, in success and children.

It's not that those things are not fulfilling; they are. They do what those things can do; they bring their own rewards: lightness and tenderness and affirmation and connection. But they don't take away the longing, the yearning, the half-conscious feeling that there is something more. And because we believe we are not enough, we also believe that if we had more or were different, we would feel nourished.

After three years of being sick, and when I was thoroughly convinced I was dying of a new, rare kind of cancer, my internist suggested that I speak to a medical intuitive, a person who diagnoses disturbances in the immune system that may be imperceptible by testing. She told me that brain surgeons and oncologists use intuitives, and that the particular one she knew had diagnosed her patients correctly ninety-eight percent of the time. Since I had already been to a spate of traditional doctors who had done nothing except mumble nonsensical diagnoses or shake their heads at my increasing weakness, I was no longer suspect of anything that sounded wooey-wooey.

I also wanted to know if I was dying.

I dialed the number.

The first thing the medical intuitive said was, "You are a control freak the likes of which I have rarely seen."

I thought about asking her if she had made a mistake, if she had switched my mother's body with mine, but I was silent.

She continued. "You wrote a book called *Breaking Free*, but you are anything but free. . . ."

I couldn't decide whether she was wild with hate or dead-on honest. I wanted to defend myself, say something witty or angry like "Bitch," but since shame, not anger, is my first reaction to being attacked (or being told the truth), I was stunned into silence.

"Most people furnish the present with thoughts of their past," she said, "but you spend all your time trying to control the future."

By this time I was looking longingly at the rug, hoping to dissolve into the cerise flower on the border. I also decided that I would never talk to my internist again.

"Imagine you have a hundred bucks to spend," she said. "Most people would spend theirs on thinking about what their parents did to them and what they regret or resent. You spend yours on fantasizing what would make you happy and then trying to orchestrate the circumstances so that they fit your fantasy. You never spend your money on the present."

She finally told me I didn't have cancer, although my immune system was "completely burned out," and that my biggest problem was that I had exhausted myself by trying to have a perfect life. She told me I had to learn to "trust and let go." (I thought: I *hate* it when people say that. Trust what? Let go of what?) She ended by telling me, "Just because you don't have cancer now doesn't

7

mean you won't have it in the future. I've seen cases where someone has developed a full-blown malignancy in forty-eight hours."

"How reassuring," I said, and we hung up.

I'd wanted answers. I'd wanted someone to tell me what was wrong with me and what to do about it. Instead she used tacky metaphors and left me more confused than when I started. Although denial and repression are not my forte, I tried to banish the conversation from my mind. Until I realized she was right. I was spending my life trying to be someone else, and even when I became the someone I thought I needed to be, I was still trying.

My first three books—*Feeding the Hungry Heart, Breaking Free,* and *Why Weight?*—focused on the descriptive and prescriptive aspects of compulsive eating: using food as an expression of unspoken needs, why diets don't work, and learning to trust the body's signals for food and satiation. *When Food Is Love* described the effect of early relationships on both eating and intimate relationships. *Appetites* takes the work a step further; it is not a book about food or body size or compulsion per se. But it *is* about true nourishment, which is also what the core obsession with thinness is about.

Women want to be thin because we believe it is a means to an end. We believe that having a thin body is the prerequisite for every other dream, and once the body is the right size, the other dreams, like dominos, can click into place, and we will at last find joy and self-value. That is a lie, but a lie upon which most women build their lives.

If she is fortunate, and if she is truthful, a woman will discover that being thin is just a body size, and she has no idea where to find true nourishment. Once she realizes it isn't in body size or success or even in loving relationships, once she slows down enough to stop defending against the emptiness, she can begin to discover what will truly feed her.

Appetites was written during a particularly difficult period in my life, a time when while some of my lifelong dreams were coming true, I was also losing what I'd never imagined I could live without—my health, my hair, my best friend. Every one of my beliefs about true nourishment was shattered in the past few years, but somewhere, between getting married and getting thin, between losing my hair and losing my best friend, I stopped believing the answer was in anything I could touch or achieve. I stopped protecting myself from the truth, stopped wishing for things to be different, and began being with myself and my life as it was. And what I discovered, in part, was that joy is actually possible—even when I am bald or sicker than I have ever been—and I keep ramrodding over it with my self-hatred and ideas of how things are supposed to be. Although I trusted that direct, consistent experiences of joy or enough-ness were possible, I thought they were reserved for people who were very holy, very wise, or very pure—which excluded me.

I was wrong. *Appetites* is a book about loss and childhood dreams and confining self-images; it is also a book about the direct experience of joy and wellness and having enough. The learnings expressed herein are not one-time learnings, but once we know what is possible, we can never go back to not knowing.

I wrote *Appetites* because I work with, and receive thousands of letters a year from, people who are hoping that if they try hard enough, their lives will match their ideas of how life is supposed to be. Like me, they think they know what needs to happen, and it's always different than what *is* happening. They, too, are tired of the fight, but they don't know what else to do.

Appetites is a book that questions our lifelong beliefs about beauty and success and friendship and the heart's desire. It is a story about what happens when we stop trying to satisfy our deepest longings with people, circumstances, or things.

In the end, this is a book about trusting and letting go. Trusting that true nourishment is available and letting go of old beliefs long enough to discover what it is.

Everything we thought was possible, is. It just doesn't look like we thought it would look, and it's not in the places we thought it would be. But it's there, it's there.

Chapter One

■

THE SIZE OF
MY BODY,
THE SIZE OF
MY LIFE

■

I'm dreaming about food again. Last night it was thick, crusty bread studded with raisins. I toasted it until it turned golden brown, then slathered it with apple butter. In my dream I picked it up, brought it slowly to my mouth, and had taken the first bite when I remembered I wasn't supposed to be eating bread. Or raisins. Or apple butter. I'm on a diet.

The last time I dreamed of food was seventeen years ago, when I was twenty-seven and on Weight Watchers. Then it was Häagen-Dazs ice cream, coffee and vanilla with hot fudge, no nuts. I dreamed of hunks of cheesecake and mountains of cookies and slabs of bittersweet chocolate. But the worst time, the time I dreamed about food every night for a year and a half, was when I was anorexic, eighteen years ago. The dreams began while I was fasting for ten days on water. It was late October and my boyfriend, Lee, and I were staying at a cabin on a lake in the Adirondacks. Every night we would go to sleep by the fire and the nubby, textiled rugs on the wall, and I would dream of feasts from college days in New Orleans: fried oysters from Casamento's, lemon doberge cake from Gambino's, napoleons from the Four Seasons on Royal Street. The sequence of the dream was always the same: I would be surrounded by food, biting down into a thick fried oyster loaf on homemade bread with pickles, horseradish, and ketchup, and suddenly my heart would pound wildly as I remembered I was supposed to be fasting. I would wrench myself awake to make sure that I hadn't really eaten the food, it was only a dream. Comforted by my abstinence, I would fall back asleep and dream of more food, more eating—and I would wake myself up again after the first bite. When I wasn't fasting, I kept myself on such a strict regime—allowing myself a hundred and fifty calories a day of raw fruits and vegetables, no protein, no fat—that my dreams were the only place I permitted myself any sweetness at all.

When I was twenty-eight, I burned my diet books in my bathtub as a symbolic statement to myself, my mother, and the world that I would never, ever diet again. Never deprive myself of foods I loved, foods I craved, foods I would not allow myself to eat except on binges. After a few months of eating ice cream every day, pizza four times a week, and croissants and chocolate chip cookies for pick-me-ups, I got the hang of it. I stopped bingeing because I stopped dieting. I realized that the fourth law of the universe is that for every diet there is an equal and opposite binge, and that if I allowed myself to eat ice cream the few times a year that

I actually wanted it, I wouldn't have to secretly, and with great shame, eat it every day.

That was sixteen years and sixty pounds ago. Since then I've written four books and taught hundreds of workshops about reaching one's natural weight without dieting.

On a national television show recently, I was speaking about the importance of allowing yourself to eat what you want; a woman in the front row began elbowing her neighbor and rolling her eyes. I lost my train of thought, and the cameras cut to a commercial for Ultra-Slim Fast.

I knew what she was thinking. She was thinking that if she let herself loose in her kitchen, she would destroy herself. She was thinking that her hunger was deep and wild, and she could devour the universe.

During the next segment I mentioned that when I tell women to eat what they want, their first reaction is either profound relief or panic. I told the story of a woman who left a workshop and bought twelve packages of Hostess Twinkies. After inhaling six of them in three minutes, she realized that they tasted awful, that she had been bingeing on them for twenty years because her mother had banned them from the house when she was twelve. "Eating what you want," I said, "frees you to discover what you *don't* want."

The woman in the first row did not snort, and I considered this a victory.

I know how difficult this is to understand. The level at which people are frightened or angry when they hear about eating what they want has nothing to do with food. It has to do with stopping the war against our-selves, the war we engage in daily when we tell ourselves that what we feel, what we want, what we look like, who we are, needs to be different. Women with food issues carry on the war through their body sizes, the food they choose to eat or not eat on a particular day, the three sizes of clothes they keep in their closets, the morning ritual of weighing in. They rage against themselves be-cause they believe that who they are is what they weigh, and what they weigh is never good enough.

It is the rage that perpetuates the suffering, not the food, not the eating, not the weight. You cannot end self-hatred with more self-hatred. You cannot learn to trust yourself by being frightened of yourself. You cannot stop the self-hatred of being fat with the self-hatred of being on a diet and depriving yourself at each meal. You can-not stop a war with another war. Eating what you want is a radical, subversive act because it stops the war.

I hadn't thought this through when I burned my diet books in the bathtub. I just wanted to stop losing and gaining ten pounds every few weeks. I wanted to stop standing at the refrigerator eating frozen cake. I wanted to stop wanting to slice off pieces of my arms and legs. Which is why I vowed never to go on another diet.

And I never have—until now.

The feelings of deprivation are as intense today as when I dreamed of fried oyster loaves. I can't eat my favorite foods: bananas in morning cereal, maple syrup on pancakes, lemon almond cookies at the end of each meal. And I can't eat chocolate. *Chocolate*. (The first time I ate a bittersweet champagne truffle, I decided that chocolate is the taste of bliss-in-matter. Chocolate is falling stars and moons and galaxies, the promise of everything you've always wanted, the seduction of unlimited possibility.) Chocolate was part of my daily maintenance program for ten years, along with flossing my teeth and taking a bath. I've explored the subtleties of Belgian, German, Swiss, French, and South American chocolate. I've experimented with malt-sweetened, fruit-juice-sweetened, unsweetened, and organic chocolate. Just a bite or two at the end of a meal gave me time to swoon, to remember that ecstasy was possible.

But a few years ago I started feeling tired all the time, and fragile, and weak. Last month I spent a week in bed with the flu, felt fine for two weeks, then was back in bed again with another virus. Like a porcelain doll that shatters, is glued back together, and shatters again, I can't seem to build up a reserve of strength or resilience before another illness knocks me down.

At first I thought I was just tired from the promotional tour for *When Food Is Love*, and decided to take a long vacation. But when I got bronchitis two weeks after returning from an island in the Pacific Northwest, I realized that something was truly wrong with my body.

I decided that I had "roving cancer" and was probably dying. After a horrible coughing spell I figured I had lung cancer. Two weeks of headaches convinced me I had a brain tumor. When I found a lump in my breast, I was certain I had breast cancer. My friends told me they were positive I was not terminally ill, but I wasn't reassured. "I'm sure Gilda Radner's friends told her the same thing," I'd say, "and her cancer started with flus and feeling weak." I was frightened that whatever was causing my ill health was momentarily dormant, coiled like a sleeping snake in the cells of my body, ready to steal my life.

During my reasonable moments I'd tell myself that I was very, very tired from constant traveling, and that four book tours and twenty workshops a year in twenty cities were finally taking their toll on my health. I'd tell myself that lightning doesn't strike in the same place twice, and since Matt's first wife died of ovarian cancer, it was not possible that God or a just universe would let his second wife die of cancer, too. I'd remember the flash of intuition I had when I was twenty-three and living in Buffalo: In the middle of a conversation with my friend Betsy about Ella, her angora cat, I suddenly knew that I was going to live until I was eighty-seven.

But at age thirty-nine I felt old and brittle, like a piece of torn rice paper. Getting out of bed each morning was a chore; walking upstairs was a major effort, and going to the movies or the store was too much to contemplate. Sometimes I thought it was all in my mind, and if only I could visualize myself being well, I'd be well. I asked myself what benefit I was receiving from being sick. I asked myself what being sick was allowing me to do that I did not allow myself when I was healthy. The answers invariably were: Rest; stay home; be still; stay quiet; retreat. So I promised myself I could stay home *and* be healthy; I cancelled a few engagements, declined invitations, and visualized myself bathed in golden light, bounding up the stairs.

Three years passed. The viruses, low-grade fevers, and chronic diarrhea got worse. I saw seventeen physicians, healers, psychics, homeopaths, chiropractors, and acupuncturists. I had blood workups, barium enemas, X rays, eye exams, ear exams, chest exams. I received diagnoses ranging from chronic fatigue syndrome to parasites; anemia to irritable bowel syndrome to hypothyroidism. I alternated between feeling hopeless about ever getting well, crazy with wondering if I had made myself sick and could therefore make myself well, and desperate for an answer to what was wrong with me.

A friend with lupus told me about Dr. Kittredge, a physician who specialized in helping people with fragile immune systems. After thoroughly questioning me about my diet and my health history, he diagnosed me with *Candida albicans*, single-cell fungi that normally live in the digestive tract. With a strong immune system, it doesn't cause a problem.

I'd known about candidiasis since a nutritionist described it to me years before. It was, she said, a condition caused by overusing antibiotics as a child or eating too many sweets or breathing too many chemicals or living on too many processed foods. She said the symptoms were fatigue, indigestion, recurring viruses, and allergies, and that the cure was following a spartan diet devoid of sweet things. I told her that everyone living in the twentieth century could have candidiasis, that it sounded like New Age hype and that any diet that eliminated sugar, and therefore chocolate, couldn't be good for the soul.

Since my encounter with the nutritionist, I've met many people who have been diagnosed with candidiasis and followed the diet. (They all, I am chagrined to say, live in California.) Some of them reported that it helped them; all of them spent the month after the diet beating a quick path to the nearest bakery, ice cream parlor, or pizza joint.

Just hearing the word *Candida* sent shivers up my spine. I thought it must have been created by a sadist, a hardened criminal who had no capacity for pleasure or sweetness except when he stole it from other people.

"How about a drug?" I say when Dr. Kittredge tells me to go on a diet of no yeast, no sweets, no dairy, no fruit, no fermented anything including mustard or vinegar or miso. I sit in his office with the photograph of sunflowers in an open field in the south of France and remember the "noir" chocolate bars I ate in Paris, the ones that were sixty-three percent chocolate, the ones I ate daily, with bread, with fruit, with cheese. I was happy then, I was healthy.

He ignores the comment. "There are many delicious things to eat besides sweets, dairy products, fruit, and bread," he says.

I am beginning to think that the cure is worse than the disease and that staying in bed with diarrhea and low-grade fevers for the rest of my life is small penance to pay for a lifetime of chocolate. I realize I am not thinking straight, am overwhelmed at the thought of not eating what I want. I still rely on food to fill in the cracks; otherwise a life without sweets wouldn't be so frightening. I stare at him. The adult voice is soon replaced by that of a three-year-old throwing a tantrum. I want to say, "Do you know who I am? I've written four books about not dieting; there is *no way* I can go on a diet. My whole life depends on my eating what I want to eat. I've staked my reputation on it."

He is busy giving me a list of delicious non-sweet things: "Steamed asparagus with lemon," he says. "Corn on the cob in the summer, butternut squash with nutmeg and cinnamon in winter. A steaming cup of jasmine tea."

"But no scones to go with the tea."

He pushes his round wire-rimmed glasses farther up his nose, brushes a piece of blond hair from his eyes, and gives me a look that says, "You just used up your self-pity-allotment." "No one is happy about this diet, Geneen, but you'll see, you'll feel better on it and you will accept it."

Since it is the week before Thanksgiving when he hands me the diet, I decide to start the Monday after Thanksgiving, a ploy I learned in my early dieting days: Decide when the diet will begin, then eat as much as you can until then. Be so sick, so bloated, so thoroughly disgusted with yourself by the time you start the diet that you will *pay* someone to remove the food from your house, so convinced are you that you will never eat again.

After I leave his office, the first thing I do is eat a handful of chocolate kisses that my friend Bari left in my car last year. I don't like milk chocolate—the kisses taste like wax, and they are beginning to catch in my throat—but I keep going, keep unwrapping, keep reaching over the passenger seat to the glove compartment to get one more. When a woman in a red Toyota honks at me because I have come within three inches of broadsiding her on one of my trans-seat maneuvers, I decide that I'm done with chocolate for the moment. A deep-dish pizza pops into my mind, stuffed with ricotta cheese and spinach and mushrooms. I haven't had pizza for a few years—cheese gives me a headache and a stuffed nose—but since I won't be allowed to have it, I want it now, tonight for dinner, tomorrow for breakfast. I am a woman on a mission, a woman on a binge.

The morning after (and for three days following) two huge pieces of Zachary's deep-dish pizza, I wake up sick, cranky, spacey. I have diarrhea for three hours and spend the rest of the day with a headache that no ibuprofen can take away. I'm getting old, I think. I used to be able to do this for two, three weeks. I take out the diet from Dr. Kittredge. Grains, vegetables, legumes, non-yeasted breads, nut butters. I decide to start immediately.

The first few days proceed smoothly. Then I start dreaming of food: cinnamon rolls, cheesecake, butterscotch pudding. When I use a Preparation H suppository for hemorrhoids that have emerged since having diarrhea, I look at it longingly, wishing it were white chocolate. I watch Matt eat an apple and get furious with how loudly he is chewing.

"Didn't your mother ever teach you to chew with your mouth closed?" I ask him.

He sighs, picks up a glass of water, and I notice, for the millionth time, that when he holds a glass, his pinkie sticks up in the air. "Poor honey," he says, "can't eat your cookies."

"Can't even eat an apple," I say, sulking.

I feel incredibly sorry for myself, disproportionately sorry. I do everything I can to convince myself that candidiasis doesn't exist. While gagging on rice with no soy sauce, morning cereal with no maple syrup, I speak to internists, family practitioners who confirm the hypothesis that being sick from yeast is New Age hype. Everyone has yeast, they acknowledge, go ahead and eat chocolate. I speak to my friend Sara, who tells me that going on the Candida diet didn't help her at all. Anna says the same thing.

Matt watches, listens to my ranting. "I don't get it," he says. "I thought this made sense to you. You've been sick for so long. Need I remind you of the barium enemas, the blood tests, the sigmoidoscopies, the rectal swabs—"

"Stop," I said. "You don't have to remind me. I remember every one of those tests. Especially the barium enema."

"None of the other doctors came up with anything after their tests except that you're exhausted and need bed rest. So why not try something that might work?"

"Because food is my issue. Take anything else away, but leave me food, especially chocolate, especially cookies."

"Yes, but don't you think that it's *because* it's your issue that it's so hard for you. Maybe it's time to do some more work. . . ."

Instead, I make an appointment with a psychic nutritionist, a woman I had heard about fifteen years ago and have always wanted to see. Theresa King lives in San Diego and comes to the Bay area twice a year to see clients. When I knock on the door of her suite at the Durant Hotel, her flaming red hair, double chin, and splashy Hawaiian muumuu greet me at the door. "Welcome," she says in an English accent, "do sit down and tell me why you've come."

As she talks to me, she checks off vegetables, meats, grains, from a long list. She puts one of her hands on my hand and sticks out her other arm in the air, keeps revolving it in circles. I wonder if her arm is cramped, needs some exercise. (Later, my friend Diane tells me that she uses her right arm as a pendulum. If, after touching my hand, her arm circles to the right when she is looking at the word asparagus, then asparagus agrees with me. If her arm circles to the left, asparagus is best left out of my diet.)

"I hope you're not a vegetarian," Theresa says as her arm swings wildly to the left.

"I am, have been one for seventeen years," I say, watching her arm.

"Dolly," she says, leaning over, putting her non-pendulum arm on my arm, "no wonder you're in such poor shape. You are protein starved. Your body wants all kinds of meat and fish. Even pork would be good for you, even eggs. You could have four ounces of beef for lunch, four for dinner."

"What about the link with high fat and breast cancer?" I ask her. "What about all the research that says that a diet high in fat isn't good for your arteries, your cholesterol, your long life?"

"Posh," she says. "People have been eating meat for centuries, and it's only been in the last few decades that cancer has become such a health issue. It's the environment, the chemicals, the pollutants that are causing cancer, not the cows. You, my dear, need meat badly."

After an hour I have a long piece of paper with a very short list of things I can eat: animal protein, broccoli, chard, Napa cabbage, oatmeal, rye, rice, and applesauce. That's it. If it isn't on the list, I can't eat it.

I promptly decide that she is crazy, that after seventeen years of being a vegetarian, I am still not willing to eat dead animals. So I make an appointment with Dr. Hamilton, another doctor who specializes in immunology. He takes twelve vials of blood from my arm, does a saliva test, a pubic hair analysis, and a stool test, and tells me that Dr. Kittredge was correct—I do have Candida. I am also allergic to beef, chicken, oatmeal, rye, chocolate, and twenty additional foods; my adrenal glands are not functioning; and I am highly allergic to molds. He prescribes fifty different supplements, a vitamin B complex shot three times a week, and a Candida diet that eliminates the foods I am allergic to as well as fermented and yeast-containing foods.

This time I am desperate. This time I am willing to do

anything to feel better. I plunge into the Candida diet with manic, religious fervor, and I start bingeing on the fifth day. Not on the usual binge foods—hunks of chocolate, slabs of raisin bread. On food that tastes like air between two pieces of cardboard. On rice crackers. On kamut bagels (don't ask). On bowls of rice puffs with rice milk. Eating when I am not hungry, not stopping when I've had enough. Making myself sick with a bloated stomach, with an empty fullness, because no matter how many bowls I eat, it is not in the nature of rice puffs (except if they are combined with butter, sugar, and marshmallows, then baked for a half hour) to produce satisfaction.

I am sorry now that I responded so casually to all those people in workshops who said, "But how can I do this when my diet is so restricted, when I have to eat a low-cholesterol diet, when I have high-blood pressure, when I have diabetes, when I am allergic to everything in the universe? How can I eat what I want and not feel deprived when I can't eat what I want and I do feel deprived?"

"There are two kinds of deprivation," I would say, "the deprivation of not eating foods you want and the deprivation of not feeling well. If you eat foods you want but don't feel well afterward, you deprive yourself of good health. You get to choose what you deprive yourself of—certain foods or well-being."

And then, with a pause and a great deal of compassion, I'd say, "The important thing to realize is that you've got a choice. You're not a victim."

Now I say: "Victim, schmictim. People who eat chocolate and raisin bread can afford to be compassionate. And smug."

It's not that I don't believe what I've said for all these years. I do. I believe that I can whine and scream, walk around feeling miserable and sorry for myself. I believe that I can act like a forty-two-year-old instead of a three-year-old, stop focusing on what I can't have, start focusing on getting well. It is my choice. It's just that as long as I whine and eat six bowls of rice puffs a day, I don't have to ask myself why, after convincing myself and the immediate world that I have a steady, sane relationship with food and my body, I am falling apart because I can't eat chocolate.

I know I am not alone. I watch the glee in people's eyes, the sparkle when dessert is brought out. The relief, and then the swoon at the first bite of sweetness. Cooing over dessert is like having a legal, public group orgasm.

My friend Josie tells me that she went on the Candida diet for three months and "it was worse than not having sex. It takes all the sensual pleasure out of food—life is too short to eat like that for too long."

My chiropractor tells me that he buys bittersweet chocolate from France in bulk at Trader Joe's and that eating it every day is "one of the greatest joys in life. I will never get my allergies tested," he says. "Never in a million years."

Marissa, my dance teacher, tells me she gained ten pounds in four months on the Candida diet because she felt so deprived that she never stopped eating. "Almond butter was my downfall," she says. "I went through three jars a week."

Anna, the receptionist in the eye doctor's office, tells me, "If you take away eating sweets from life, there's not a lot left to look forward to. I know that sounds absurd—I love my life, my job, my kids, my husband. But food—that's a whole different story."

My colleague Lizzie says, "For me, it's my two glasses of wine at dinner and some kind of sweet every day. I look forward to that wine all day long; it makes me so happy to be sitting there, sipping, going over the day, relaxing. I don't know what I would do if I had to stop drinking, and at the same time I know that someday I will have to because I am too dependent on it and that is disturbing."

Even Dean Ornish, the proponent of the lower-than-low-fat diet, says, "I wouldn't be happy in a world without chocolate."

I console myself with the fact that other people are as attached to what brings them sweetness as I am. Everyone seems to have their own little pocket of pleasure, some kind of food or drink they rely on to get them through a day. I do not believe that these familiar comforts are bad or that we have to give them up. I do not believe in deprivation for its own sake or to prove a point. There is joy in familiar comforts, and anything that can bring us joy and pleasure has value.

It's not the joy and pleasure that causes trouble, of course—it's the attachment to it, the identification with it.

My cousin Judith used to spend ten minutes each morning making her morning brew: leaves of Earl Grey tea steeped for four minutes. While the tea was steeping, she'd take her favorite mug, add two spoonfuls of sugar and a quarter cup of hot milk. Not boiled or scalded, just heated enough for bubbles to begin forming around the edges. The milk had to be added to the mug before the tea, the sugar before the milk, or the mixture was ruined. Then her doctor told her that caffeine was causing cysts in her breasts and that milk was making her arthritis worse. After considering the alternatives for a few days, Judith decided that she would rather have cysts and arthritis than mornings without tea.

We create rituals, rely on substances that not only bring us pleasure but make us feel safe. Then we feel as if we cannot live without them. It happens slowly. We turn what brings us pleasure into what eventually protects us from feeling more pleasure (i.e., the pleasure that comes from being healthy). We tighten ourselves around a particular way of eating or looking or relating and believe that (being thin, being a non-dieter, being a writer, being a mother, being a lawyer, being single) is what we need. We fix our identities on being and having certain things and believe that letting go of them means losing who we are.

I heard a tape by a doctor recently in which she said that it's not unusual for someone with cancer to be confronted with the choice of giving up cigarettes or dying, and to choose the cigarettes. And although it is true that nicotine is addictive, it is also true that it is terrifying to go unprotected, even in our own house. Not to define ourselves by what we look like, what we eat, what we do, what our children do. And yet when we believe we have to have, look like, or be a particular thing, we close ourselves to the possibility of change. We make the assumption that who we are today is who we will be tomorrow, and that what we needed last year is what we need today. If we give up what we needed last year, we believe we will lose everything that could bring us happiness tomorrow.

What happens when we have to let go of something we never thought we could let go of?

D. T. Suzuki, the teacher who brought Zen to America, said, "In the beginner's mind, there are many possibilities; in the expert's mind, there are few."

When you are full of what you know, it's difficult to learn anything new.

Three weeks have passed. I am still leaving a trail of rice in every room, find myself bending down and picking up smashed puffs on the way to the bathroom, the living room, my study. But something has shifted. I don't miss the taste of sweetness; I miss *the idea* of it. Last week Matt and I were buying cinnamon dental floss in Bill's Drugs, and their Valentine's candy was on sale. Four rows deep of pink and gold and red cardboard hearts festooned with ribbons and bows and plastic flowers. As we passed the last box, I was suddenly seized with a desire to hide behind the L'eggs panty hose until the store closed and then to tear open the boxes, sit in the middle of the aisle, and eat every single light green-filled chocolate in box after tacky box. When morning came, my skin would be green like the inside of the chocolates, I would be dazed and burping, beached in the aisle like a baby whale, but I would be fortunate to be in a drugstore, where the pharmacist would know what to do.

We stood in the check-out line behind a six- or seven-year-old girl with straight blond hair and a red-and-white-striped headband. She pulled on her mother, who was ignoring her, as she tried to pay for the cat food and toilet paper. Can't I, Mom, the girl pleaded, can't I just have a little chocolate heart? Just that little one? She pointed at the display behind us, and I looked to see which one had captured her fancy. A red See's candy box wrapped in cellophane. Bad choice, I thought. Looks like it has caramels and liquid centers. I'd go for the gold one behind it. In my experience, gold boxes usually contain solid chocolate rounds wrapped in colored foil.

The mother, who was clearly exasperated, said, "I've told you a million times. The doctor says you can't have chocolate after dinner. Here, I'll buy you some chewing gum." She reached for a package of Trident gum, original flavor, in the blue package.

The girl looked at the gum and then back at the chocolate heart. She knew that accepting gum for chocolate was at best a poor second, and at worst a trick, but she took it anyway. Even artificial sweetness is better than none.

We paid for our purchase and left. "At least the dental floss is sweet," I said to Matt as we walked to our car.

"Oh, honey," he said, putting the key in the car door, "you really have it bad."

"Yeah," I murmured as I glanced back at the store for a corner of a heart, a glint of a plastic flower. "I certainly do."

I miss the freedom of being able to choose what I want to eat, and consequently I am bingeing because I'm supposed to be dieting. Since nut butters are permissible foods, I dive into jars of cashew, sesame, almond, macadamia, pistachio, and pecan butter a few times a day. Heaping tablespoonfuls, one after the other. Sometimes I stop to spread it on rice crackers, but most times, because rice crackers are so crumbly and take time to unwrap, I skip the intermediate step and head directly for the mouth. And, as anyone who eats a half jar of nut butter a day would, I am gaining weight. My thighs are beginning to rub together as they used to, my pants are getting tight, my stomach is sticking out.

Despite all this I am actually feeling better. I wake up in the morning and I want to get out of bed. Once out of bed, I have energy to walk up the stairs. After meditating and eating breakfast, I want to write, speak to friends, take a walk instead of crawling back under the covers. The sun is out in my body again. It's as if I have a bottom to myself, as if I am filling up instead of forever emptying out.

A person would think—it makes obvious sense—that feeling better would ease the deprivation, would inspire me to follow the diet cheerfully, to lie down and kiss the earth in gratitude. Wrong. I am thrilled to be given the chance at well-being again. But it's not like having a near-death experience and upon return never taking the color blue for granted again. It's subtle, it's slow—I still have many moments of feeling ragged and fragile—and food was my issue. Is my issue. Will always be my issue (or at least one of my issues. Issues are something about which I feel abundant).

I am trying to be reasonable. I am trying not to panic at the incipient double chin. I am telling myself that this is not forever and that in a few months the doctor said I can begin adding more foods, although, he added, noticing the hopeful gleam in my eye, chocolate will not be one of them. On days when the self-talk works, I am reassured, I feel like an adult. I even manage to wait until I am hungry to eat the next three bowls of rice puffs, vegetable glycerine, and unsweetened carob powder. But then something happens—I get some good news or some bad news. Matt sneezes, Erica and Dimitri have a fight on *All My Children*, and before you can say sesame tahini, I am spooning it into my mouth. Afterward, I am frightened that I will gain fifty pounds, that everything I have worked so hard to become is a sham because after a sixteen-year hiatus, I am dieting and bingeing and gaining weight again.

I wish this weren't so. I wish I could act like an adult instead of a three-year-old when I am told not to eat chocolate because it makes me sick. I wish getting better was enough of a reward. I wish I could be on this diet without bingeing, but most of all, I wish it didn't matter so much that I am gaining weight. I thought I was over that.

When I first stopped dieting, I was terrified by the possibility that I would gain weight until I was fatter than I had ever been, fatter than I ever imagined myself being. I had no idea if eating what I wanted would mean eating a half gallon of vanilla fudge twirl ice cream, three pieces of chocolate cake, and a loaf of raisin bread slathered with butter every day for fifty years, and since I blamed every love lost and every setback, every disappointment and every frustration on my weight from the time I was four to the present moment, the possibility of being fat sent me into a raw, primal panic. My heart would beat fast, I'd start to sweat, and my words would get jammed together. I'd feel as if I was about to walk off a cliff, land in a foreign country, and have to start over again with a new language, new relationships, new definitions of love and beauty. But I was willing. I was willing to be fat for the rest of my life if it meant I stopped loathing myself. If I could stop walking around feeling like a crazed, feral animal who was ready to eat the refrigerator as soon as no one was looking, I was willing to do anything. Even be fat.

I never had to test my convictions, not really. Because although I was fifty pounds overweight when I started, and although I subsequently gained ten pounds, I started to lose weight within six months and continued to get thinner over the years.

And it's not as if I really believe that now, when I am eating nut butter by the tablespoonful, I will gain a hundred pounds. I don't believe I will ever be fat. But neither do I believe that it is possible for me, given my basically round body, to stay as thin as I've been for ten years. And that is sending me into the same word-jamming, heart-beating paroxysm of fear that I was thrown into years ago.

Because not being thin feels the same as being fat. My friend Natalie once told me that she was disappointed by life. "It's not that I don't have many moments of happiness," she said. "It's just that I thought there was going to be a big victory, and there is none. Life just keeps going on and on."

For me, being thin was the big victory. Different from writing books, teaching workshops, getting married to a man I love. Different from walking in a thousand-year-old redwood forest, watching the sun streak into the ocean, swimming with dolphins. All of those are in one category, and being thin is in another. Being thin is a category of its own.

I am living two lives. One life, the life I show to the world, is passionate about, and deeply involved with, friends, family, work. The other life, the one I don't talk about, is passionate about one thing only: being and staying thin.

Last year my friend Marina, who had to take the drug prednisone for Krohn's disease and gained thirty-five pounds in the process, told me she would give her right pinkie to be thin again.

I said, "Listen to yourself. You sound like a crazy person, like a woman who has no value except in the shape of your body."

She said, "You try being thin and then gaining thirty-five pounds, and we'll see how you like it. We'll see what you are willing to do to have your teeny tiny body back again."

We were sitting in another friend's living room at the time of our talk. The table behind Marina was lined with family photographs, each one framed in silver: a little girl with a wreath of flowers around her head dressed in a long purple velvet dress; a couple getting married, the bride wearing a long white dress glittering with sequins. I remember that when Marina said the words "teeny tiny," I was looking at the sequins of the wedding dress, and despite the tone of the conversation, a flush of pleasure spread across my chest. The justification, the validation, the victory of at long last being perceived as thin. ("Being thin is so temporary," my friend Deborah remarks. She weighs ninety-five pounds, was a skinny child, but had a seven-year cycle twenty years ago when she gained fifty pounds and struggled to take it off. Now, despite the fact that she's been the same weight for many years, she feels as if being thin is temporary and at any moment she could get fat.)

My father ate rows of Fig Newtons at one sitting and didn't gain weight. My brother drank Yoo-Hoo chocolate milk followed by Ring-Dings and Tastee doughnuts and stayed lean. My mother, trained by her mother before her, and I, carrying the legacy, labored like sea turtles under the burden of a "weight problem." We watched the boys eat their high-calorie treats as we surrounded ourselves with carrot sticks and melba toast and No-Cal coffee soda. In the kitchen before holidays, we appeared, my mother, my grandmother, my cousin, and me, to eat the rugalah, the potato pancakes, the matzo balls, the macaroons, that we wouldn't allow ourselves to eat in full view of the family. It wasn't a purposeful gathering; it was a one-at-a-time swipe at a potato pancake when no one was looking, a grab for a cookie when we were clearing the dishes. Stuffing it in our mouths while pretending to be doing something else. Stealing moments to eat stolen food. But it was the only way to have what the boys were given for free. If we ate anything fattening in front of anyone—especially each other—it meant we were satisfied with the shape of our bodies, that we had the audacity to be content despite the fact that we weren't as thin as we could be. Ought to be. Needed to be.

I won.

I did what they told me I couldn't do: I got thin. And I did it by eating what they told me I couldn't eat: chocolate.

It is December of last year and I have the flu. I am so sick that I cannot lift my head. My temperature keeps rising—one day it is a hundred and two, the next day, a hundred and four. Matt holds me in the middle of the night when I wake up shivering, tells me stories about people in a strange land who have walnut shells attached to their fingernails on which they write whole books. They even have little toasters in the shells, he whispers at three a.m., and people give out pieces of toast to celebrate finishing a book. Do they put strawberry jam on the toast, I ask him, and then feel sick to my stomach at the thought of food? No, he says, only walnut butter and only to people who don't have the flu. He continues the story night after middle of the night through the shivering and the soaked sheets. After ten days of drinking broth, my bones are beginning to stick out of my chest. As sick as I am, I like the feeling of fragility, of getting smaller and smaller. I manage to get out of bed on the fifth day to try on a pair of leggings I bought a few years ago that have since gotten too tight. Now they hang shapelessly, and I smile for the first time in days. When I crawl out of bed to go to the bathroom each morning, I put my hand on my stomach to see how flat it is getting, lift up my nightgown while I stand in front of the mirror to see how thin I look. With each rib bone I see, a bird of gladness flies from my heart.

Three weeks later, I am shown into my doctor's office for my yearly physical and asked to undress, put on a blue cotton gown. I get on the scale and see that I weigh a hundred pounds. I haven't been this thin since I was anorexic, when I weighed eighty-two.

The doctor comes in, checks my reflexes, listens to my lungs, takes a pap smear. She asks me to get on the scale.

I already did, I say. I weigh a hundred pounds.

She looks at my bony arms, chest, my gaunt face. Can I believe you? she asks.

What do you mean? I say.

Some of my anorexic patients put rocks in their pockets to weigh more than they do.

No rocks, I answer, smiling in disbelief. I can't believe she thinks I would actually lie about my weight. That was something I used to do when I was fifteen (and more recently, on driver's licenses and insurance applications). But it was always underestimating my weight. She thinks I am overestimating. I must look really thin. Another bird soars from my heart.

Now it is March and I am gaining weight on the Candida diet. This morning I tried on my loose jeans, and they are snug around the waist, the thighs. I feel my belly when I wake up, hoping to find it flat but knowing, after five bowls of rice puffs and a half jar of cashew butter, it won't be.

Being thin was the magic that was supposed to heal the damage at the core of me, the damage symbolized by fat. If I lost the weight, I'd lose the damaged core. And although being thin did not do what I thought it would, I still believe in its magic. Of all the familiar comforts of my life, being thin is the one that remains constant. And although I feel loved and seen by everyone who matters to me, with each bite of cashew butter, the panic rises into a familiar hysteria. With each bite I come closer and closer to the fat and clumsy eight-year-old with hair that wouldn't flip and a mother who wouldn't stay.

I know what I have to do, and I don't want to do it.

I have to be willing to gain weight. More precisely, I have to be willing to accept the weight I am already gaining. Fifteen pounds, twenty. I might not gain that much, but I need to be willing to, because it is the open-handed, tender-hearted willingness (the *love*, the *love*) that melts the rock of fear wedged in my bones. I have to be willing to have a bigger body than every part of me screams I should, and remind myself (this time, next time, the time after that) that I am still allowed, still entitled, still deserve to respect myself, even cherish myself. I don't have to be small to be big. But neither do I have to be big to be big. I only have to be the size I am, whatever that is in a given moment, at a given time in my life.

The question is: How do I know what size I am supposed to be? Is it the size I reach after bingeing on jars of nut butter for six weeks? Is it the size I would reach by eating nut butter and not bingeing? Or is it the size I was before I started eating nut butter, the size I have been, give or take a few pounds, for ten years?

Perhaps there is no size I am supposed to be. Perhaps what is important is not the size, not the weight, but the life I lead as I am getting there, being there. If, while I am bingeing on cashew butter and rice in every form, I lead a life of integrity and passion, why would being thin matter so much? Isn't it the associations I have with gaining weight, rather than the weight itself, that are so painful? Isn't it the connection I want anyway? The ability to participate fully in life today, this very moment, instead of waiting for some magical future time when I will have fulfilled all the requirements and be good enough to be alive? Isn't that the reason I want to be thin—because I believe that being thin and being worthy are synonymous?

It is not the size of my body I care so passionately about, but the size of my life. But the two are so inexorably tangled together, like skeins of wool knotted in ten thousand places, that it is almost impossible to take them apart, to truly comprehend that, no matter what this culture would have us believe, they are separate.

The belief around which all other beliefs are clustered is that the size of my body determines the size of my life. I have been living with that belief for so many years that it's become the ground I walk on. I don't think about it, don't question it. I just walk. But if I engage in the subversive act of untangling the body threads from the life threads, I find the bare truths of a lifetime:

My mother would have felt trapped and incapable of generous love whether I weighed eighty or a hundred and sixty pounds.

I have been loved passionately and tenderly at a hundred and sixty pounds. My weight has made no difference in the quality of love in my life. Ever.

I have loathed myself at a hundred and ten pounds and cherished myself at a hundred and sixty.

Being thin gives me what size can give me: a lighter body, greater ease of movement, smaller clothes, cultural acknowledgment. That's all, that's it.

These are not one-time epiphanies. They are threads that will get tangled again and again. And the only way I know to live with that knowledge is to keep walking into the fear of being fat, to keep uncovering my beliefs about being thin—and to be willing to gain weight. And to do the whole process over and over, as many times as it takes, from now until I walk on different ground or I am reborn in Samoa (where a woman is not considered attractive unless she weighs two hundred pounds).

There isn't an end to this issue. Or to any other core issue. You think you have it all fixed—your weight is stable, you have the eating thing down, life is good—and then your best friend is diagnosed with AIDS or your house collapses in an earthquake or you're told you can't eat chocolate. And it starts again.

For thirty years I have been coming around and around on the spiral of being thin, and each time it is the same, and each time it is different. My friend Molly, a recovering alcoholic and an ex-bulimic, says that, like alcoholism, compulsive eating is a disease from which you never fully recover. I don't agree with her. Even now, when I am drowning in six kinds of nut butters, I don't believe that this is a disease. Diseases are relative. Someone is sick compared to someone who is not sick; there has to be health for sickness to exist. If compulsive eating is a disease, there is no one who is not sick. The whole culture has the same disease. The whole culture believes that being thin makes a woman worthy and being fat makes her a failure.

In a recent survey in *Esquire* magazine, a thousand women were asked whether they would rather be run over by a truck or gain a hundred and fifty pounds. Fifty-four point three percent answered that they would rather be run over by a truck. That means that they would rather be paralyzed for the rest of their lives than gain weight. They would rather be brain dead than gain weight. They would rather lose an arm, a leg, a kidney, an eye, than gain weight. Fifty-four point three percent of the women surveyed would rather risk death than gain weight. Because the size of their bodies determines the quality of their lives, they would rather be dead than be fat.

There isn't an end to dealing with the longing to be thinner than you are. If the truth is that you'd rather be run over by a truck than be fat, it's crucial to say that, to know that, because you can move from there. You can feel the utter depravity of being in a culture that values being thin more than being alive, and you can ask yourself how you are going to live with that prejudice, what you are going to do about it. You can work with it, speak up about it. Tell your daughter that she is beautiful no matter what.

There isn't an end. There isn't a cure. There is only a relationship and the willingness to enter into it every time it calls you. To look and see how you identify yourself, where you find safety. Are you your body? Does your life depend on being thin? Does your experience of pleasure depend on eating chocolate? Because if you are, and if it does, your identity and safety are as fragile as mine were.

I thought I had handled the eating thing. Which was true—as long as I was healthy, could eat what I wanted, could weigh what I weighed. As long as I could carry bags of lemon almond cookies, poppyseed muffins, and bittersweet chocolate on the plane, as long as I was as thin as I wanted to be, I was safe. I knew who I was.

But I can't eat chocolate and I'm gaining weight, and I have to discover what is real again when I am not adorning myself with delicious foods, a thin body, and the protective armor of someone who has solved her weight problem.

Because I can't rely on having the body I want or eating foods I want, the question of who I am without those things ripples through my heart. On what does my life depend? What is it that gets me out of bed every morning?

I thought I had arrived at the answers years ago. But I am still arriving. For many years the motivation to work through the obsession with food drove my days. Fueled my work. Gave me an identity. Falling in love added a new passion and a new identity: I was someone's partner, then someone's wife. Layers of safety, of being Someone. Gaining weight, and being willing to gain more, makes everything new again. Cleans the slate.

Food and eating are my lifelong issues. And my lifelong teachers. Because they cause me immeasurable pain, they open the door to immeasurable richness. Because I cannot answer my need for sweetness with food, because I cannot spend the meal anticipating the cookie at the end of the meal, I remain in the present more of the time. And I allow myself sweetness in other places: the buttery yellow ranunculas; the mourning dove who takes a bath in the saucer of water on my deck; roasting pumpkin seeds; the tangerine smell of Matt's skin; Blanche's gurgling purr.

When I walked into the Berkeley Rose Garden yesterday and saw the flowers wide open and unafraid to be gorgeous, the fog rolling above the Golden Gate Bridge, the bay shimmering with light, I felt as if I was suspended between beliefs. For a few moments the fact that I could see and hear and breathe and walk, that lushness and light and shameless beauty existed in such profusion, seemed miraculous. I stood next to the Blue Nile roses and watched the sun slide behind the bay.

Then I walked to Bill's Drugs for a bottle of hydrogen peroxide (Dr. Hamilton says I am allergic to mold and that hydrogen peroxide kills the green clumps growing on my windowsill). I passed Hillary Heffelflopper on my way to aisle 3B. Her ears were pointed, her eyes were buttons of white and blue candy. Her long body, of course, was made of chocolate. Milk, not bittersweet. Hollow, not solid. Next to her on the shelf was Harold Heffelflopper, wearing chocolate suspenders, and next to him, Just Born Peeps, a package of thirty-six neon green and pink marshmallow chicks waiting to be discovered in a child's basket of cellophane grass and painted eggs. The packages of Hugs was the attention grabber, though. Hershey's kisses hugged in a layer of white chocolate. I sighed, I salivated, and then I remembered the rose garden.

Flanked by Hillary and Harold, I asked myself if I would give up a lifetime of chocolate for a lifetime of moments like those in the rose garden.

In a second, I answered.

But would you give up a lifetime of being thin? I asked myself.

These questions are ridiculous, I said out loud, and quickly looked around to see if anyone had heard. They reminded me of the day my friend Fleur called and said, "If you had to give up hot water or sex for the rest of your life, which would you give up?"

"Does giving up hot water mean that I couldn't have tea or tepid baths?" I asked.

"Not one hot water bottle, bath, cup of tea, steam room," she answered. "Nothing that depends on or is made of hot water."

"I hate to say this, Matt would not be happy if he knew, but I'd give up sex. I'd be cold so much of the time that taking my clothes off would be impossible."

"Me too," she answered. "Now, I have another question. If you had to give up hot water or laughter for the rest of your life, which would you give up?"

"This is ridiculous," I answered. "It's never going to come to that."

"Answer the question," she said.

"Well," I drawled, "hot water is good for my body, but I can't imagine living without laughter, wouldn't want to. Without laughter I wouldn't even care about hot water."

Standing in a pasture of pastel and milk chocolate, I realize the questions about hot water and being thin are the same. One choice is about valuing my body above all else; the other is about valuing the spirit that animates my body.

Would I give up being thin for the possibility of not armoring myself, not separating myself from roses, suffering, passion, other people? Would I give up the comfort of knowing who I am and fitting in for not knowing and being willing to unfold myself day by day?

In an instant, I answered, and sashayed past the dental floss and suppositories on my way to the hydrogen peroxide.

Chapter Two

■

THE HUNGER TO
BE VALUED

■

I never told anyone I wanted to be famous until I was thirty-nine, which meant I'd been living with the secret for thirty-one years. It wasn't the kind of thing I revealed when asked what I wanted to be when I grew up. I was embarrassed by it, even at eight years old. Embarrassed by the grandness of it, the fact that I dared to dream in such a large size.

My friends seemed to dream on a smaller scale (or else they, too, wanted to be famous and didn't tell). They said they wanted to be doctors, lawyers, artists, or wives of doctors, lawyers, and artists. For a brief moment I considered being a doctor, but mostly I wanted to be famous in a huge, silvery way.

Matt was the first person I told, but by then I was well into my fourth book and had attached the fame part to the book part.

In reality, they are separate. My writing has nothing to do with wanting to be famous; it is a way to ground myself in my own life, to connect with the lives of other people. But since I have no acting talent and do not look like a model, and since I have no desire to be a talk-show host or do anything else that could generate fame, I used what I had to get what I wanted.

Writers become famous when, for one reason or other, their books hit the *New York Times* bestseller list. To get and stay "on the list," a book has to sell as many or more copies in a given week than the other books on that list. Which means letting as many people as possible know— within the shortest given time—that your book is in the stores. Which means interviews on television and radio and newspaper, as many as eight or nine a day.

In addition to the national shows, there is also the belief that if you work very hard, if you never turn down an interview, if you spend eighty percent of your time publicizing your book on any television show anywhere, if you visualize success and if you never give up, you can have a bestselling book.

My friend Ken Blanchard, co-author of *The One Minute Manager*, a *New York Times* bestseller for two years, coached me on the steps to literary fame. "Cut out the *Times* list and paste it where you can see it. Imagine your book climbing from number ten to number three to number one. Make phone calls every day to people who might be able to help you. Speak to the retailers, the wholesalers, the distributors; speak to the sales force at your company. You've got to want it badly," he told me.

Before her first book, *How to Make Love All the Time*, became a bestseller, I received a postcard from Barbara De Angelis, explaining that it was her dream to be on the *New York Times* list, and she was asking all her friends, associates, and fans to buy her book the same day. The huge volume of sales at one time would, she hoped, place the book on the list. When I read her card, I was astonished by her honesty and chutzpah; she made herself so vulnerable. My theory had always been: If you don't tell anyone what you want, you don't have to be embarrassed when you don't get it.

At summer camp when I was thirteen, I had a crush on Josh Goldstein. One day he was standing on a big white rock (we called it "the wishing rock"), and I was walking in the meadow below. He motioned to me to follow him to the basketball court. I would have followed him any-where, but I didn't want to let him know that, so I crossed my arms, gave him a coy, seductive smile, and stayed where I was. He shrugged his shoulders, and said, "Okay, but don't say I didn't give you a chance." The next day he asked my best friend, Joanie Newhouse, to go steady with him. She said yes, and wore his silver ID bracelet for the rest of the summer.

There are many ways to interpret this story. One is: Thank God I found out what a schmuck Josh was before it was too late. Another is: When your best friend goes steady with your heartthrob, she really isn't your best friend. Still another is: Carpe diem; if you don't go after what you want, someone else will. Be like a tiger and charge.

Twenty-six years later, I charged. I gave myself entirely

to the task of becoming famous with the publication of *When Food Is Love.* I went on a thirty-city book tour; I taught twenty workshops in different cities along the tour; I agreed to every interview, every book signing, every appearance, even if it meant criss-crossing the country a few times a week. I cut out the bestseller list; I visualized; I affirmed.

It is Monday of last week; Matt and I are shopping for groceries at Living Foods. I look like I usually look— rumpled, with glow-in-the-dark sweat pants, a sweater big enough for three, and a baseball cap. While I am picking out a Crenshaw melon, the woman behind the deli counter says to Matt, "Are you Matt?"

He says, "That's me."

"I know all about you . . ."

I hear bits of the conversation as I push the center of the third melon. Someone's recognized Matt, I think. Someone has been to one of his talks, that's nice. He likes that. When he comes back I ask, "Has she been to one of your talks?"

"No," he replies, "she's read all your books. She recognized your face and figured I was the guy you write about. She loves your work. She says it changed her life."

I feel a combination of pleasure and fear shimmy up my back. Pleasure because the book is actually reaching people. People such as the woman behind the deli counter in my local grocery store are willingly (not because they are my friends and they have to) reading it and being affected by it. That makes me extraordinarily happy.

Fear because I am suddenly not an anonymous person pressing melons. The woman behind the deli counter has an idea of who she thinks I am, of who she wants me to be, based on her reading of the book, and there is no way I can match her idea. Not with my dirty hair, crankiness, and sheen of white cat fur covering my clothes. Not with the way I feel about myself today—uncertain, depressed, and generally miserable. Today I feel like I must have been on drugs when I decided to write another book. Today I worked on one paragraph for seven hours, after which I threw it in the garbage. Today I had a fight with Matt, missed my appointment with the accountant, forgot my mother's birthday. Today I can't remember anything good or kind or decent about myself. I certainly cannot relate to or identify with writing a book that someone actually liked.

The woman walks over to me, a broad smile on her face. I consider telling her that Matt was joking, that I did not write any books, and she is mistaking me for someone else. I quickly decide that this would be a violation of the fourth precept that I took with Thich Nhat Hanh, the one about not lying, and so I don't.

"I don't mean to bother you," she says. "I know you came here to shop, but I just have to tell you what your books mean to me."

I smile my best smile, and wonder if the piece of Swiss chard from dinner is still stuck in my front tooth. I notice that I'm not hearing anything she is saying. I am too busy putting up walls, thinking that she wants something I can't give her, that she thinks I am better than I know I am.

". . . and so I keep your book by my bed and read it when I need to remember that I am fine just the way I am. Thank you." She takes my hand, touches it gently, then walks back to the deli.

I stare at the intricate lace patterns on her skirt as she walks away. She didn't want to take anything from you, a voice in my head says. She wanted to give something to you, and you missed it because you were so afraid of being robbed of your misery.

I wheel the cart down the frozen-foods aisle, take two bags of strawberries, a bag of cherries from the freezer. Why did I want to be famous? What did I think it would feel like to be recognized by someone I didn't know?

I didn't think. It never occurred to me that anyone would stop me in a store, want to talk to me on the street. I wanted the whole world to know my face, my name, but I never actually thought about going to the grocery store. I never realized that "the whole world" was made up of individual people in grocery stores and airports. I wanted to be wanted by people *I knew* didn't want me, not people I didn't know. It never occurred to me that a stranger would recognize my face (even though it's plastered on the covers of four books). Or that she would want to talk to me when I look like an unmade bed. It never occurred to me that people would idealize me the same way I idealize Toni Morrison or Deena Metzger.

In a recent workshop, three or four women stood up and said they thought I was a goddess. I said, "Hey, girls, this is a serious misunderstanding. I know what it feels like to be inside my body, and believe me, you wouldn't want to be here most of the time." I gave them concrete examples: how I had acted like a three-year-old with Matt that morning, how stingy I had been with my friend Leslie last week. They shrugged. So what, they said, you're still a goddess.

I told them about the women I'd met on a TV show the previous week, all television stars, all with eating disorders. One of them described how she starved herself for four days each week, then spent the remaining three days eating tens of thousands of calories, after which she threw up everything. Between binges she took hormone shots and posed for the cover of teen magazines. Gave diet tips. A bulimic taking hormone shots, consumed with self-loathing, was giving diet tips to teenage girls.

Yeah, but that was the television star, they said to me. You're not eating and throwing up. You're not pretending to be someone you're not. It doesn't make us think less of you when you tell us you act like a three-year-old. It makes us think more of you because you have the guts to say it.

Yes, I said, but where does this end? If I see Toni Morrison as a goddess and you see me as a goddess, isn't it just our need to see goddesses that we are dealing with?

This year, four years after the publication of *When Food Is Love*, Barbara Walters interviewed Jim Carrey, star of *The Mask*, who told her that ten years ago, when he was unknown in Hollywood, he had drafted himself a check for ten million dollars. In the memo space on the check, he wrote, "for acting services rendered." He carried the check in his wallet, allowing it to be a reminder of his luminous dreams. At night he drove up to Mulholland Drive, where the movie stars lived, and imagined himself living like one of them. Imagined the life he was leading, the ballrooms he was walking through, the elegance, the fame. When he was thoroughly convinced that he was accomplished and famous and rich, he drove back to his small apartment.

The reason, of course, Barbara Walters was interviewing him was that he had just signed a contract for ten million dollars for acting services rendered, and he was now living the life of the rich and famous residents of Mulholland Drive.

As I listened to him, I couldn't decide whether he was a fabulous example of the power of affirmation and positive thinking, or whether fame-hungry people would hear his words, believe that they, too, could be famous, write multimillion-dollar checks to themselves, and spend their evenings staring at mansions on hills.

Listening to him made me want to write a check to myself, puff up my chest, and go back into the world of Trying-to-Be-Famous because although the book actually made it on the *Times* list for two weeks, I never achieved the silvery fame I yearned for. Carrey's interview reminded me of the distance between what was possible and what had happened, and it brought up my questions again. Was I not talented enough as a writer? Did I not try hard enough? Does trying have anything to do with it, or is it fate, destiny, karma, luck?

And there was the issue of fame itself. Why did I want to be famous, anyway? It is possible to teach, write, and want my work to reach people without wanting to be famous. In Buddhism, desire is the root of all suffering; the desire to be famous is nothing more than an indication of being seduced by the belief that the temptations of the world can make me happy. Or, as Annie Lamott says, "If the world thinks it's great, it's probably lined with cocaine."

Before the publication of the book, a Buddhist friend called and said, "I hope it reaches millions of people. I hope everyone who reads it is helped tremendously. I hope it goes a long way to stop suffering. And I hope that despite it all, you never get rich and famous because that would only add to your suffering."

I knew he was right. I knew that fame was not the answer. I had been through this a hundred times. The "When I Am Famous" dream was the "When I Am Thin" rap transferred to bestsellerdom. It was the syncopated beat of "When I Fall in Love and Meet the Man of My Dreams" mixed with the tunes of "When We Live in the Country" and "When I Have That Dress I Saw Today." I know they are longings that replace other, more elusive longings, and, earnest as they are, they can never satisfy what they are intended to replace.

Knowing that hasn't stopped me, though. It didn't stop me from wanting to be thin, and it didn't stop me from believing that when I met Matt, I would be forever happy, and it didn't stop me from throwing myself into trying to be famous. The longing is so old and has gone unrecognized for so many years that it has a life of its own. It thinks it's about whatever I don't have.

Being on the *Times* list was glorious for two entire days. Then I started obsessing about staying on it. Two weeks later, the *Rand McNally Road Atlas* replaced *When Food Is Love* on the list, and I was crushed.

Thirty-one years of wild wanting for forty-eight hours of happiness.

I'm not a good Buddhist, that's clear. It's not enough for me to know about the wanting mind. It's not enough to know that the nature of mind is to want whatever it doesn't have, and that everyone's mind does the same thing. It's not enough to know that being famous will not make me happy. I still want to be famous.

It is the same dilemma that women in my workshops face with the desire to be thin. Every one of them knows, because most of them have already experienced it, that being thin will not satisfy the longing in their hearts, yet they continue their wild wanting year after year. If they are not dieting and bingeing, if their weight is not actually going up and down, they are obsessed with staying thin. With exercising or no-fat diets or the fear of what will happen if they gain weight.

And it is the same dilemma that anyone faces when a goal is reached, when a dream is realized—being promoted or falling in love or living in the country or buying the dress you saw today. Every time we do something, dream something, achieve something that we think is going to fix what is wrong, every time we do it for what it will bring us rather than for joy of the act itself, disappointment is inevitable. But rather than allow the pain of this, we switch to the next dream. A bigger car, a smaller body, a different job, more fame.

There are four shelves of breads at Living Foods, an entire wall. Endless varieties of hamburger rolls, hot dog rolls, twelve kinds of wheat bread. I look for the Tassajara Onion Dill bread with the blue writing, sort through the Vital Vittles Three Seed, Sesame-Millet, Cornbread, Sourdough Rye. No Tassajara Dill. I keep moving.

I thought I wanted to be a person Barbara Walters would want to interview.

I thought I wanted to leave people dazzled and in awe of me. I was wrong.

I thought that if enough people wanted to be me, I would want to be myself. I was wrong about that, too. Because when someone looks at me with stars in her eyes, as if I have the answer to her pain or am better than she is, I want to tell her that I don't have the answers, and that there is a long distance between who she thinks I am and who I know I am.

It's not fame I wanted. I wanted to rest, to stop the relentless push to be someone I didn't think I was, to get something I didn't think I had. I thought being famous would give that to me. I thought being famous would be about being seen and being wanted and being loved in gigantic, undeniable, irresistible ways.

I am face to face with the nut butters. The organic peanut butter is on sale, $2.89 for a jar. My boyfriend David used to make peanut butter, mayonnaise, and lettuce sandwiches in Buffalo twenty years ago. We'd spread a red-checkered cloth on the gold and black Indian print-covered couch, arrange the peanut butter sandwiches, Cokes and Pepperidge Farm Lido cookies in an elegant arrangement and sprawl into the snowy afternoons, feeding each other. Besides its unusual taste, the good thing about mixing peanut butter with mayonnaise is that it doesn't stick to the roof of your mouth or get caught in your throat, which makes it possible to talk while lying down. With his head in my lap, David would muse about teaching D. H. Lawrence to college students, and I would muse about meeting Joni Mitchell, my goddess of the moment. Although I didn't say it out loud, I wanted what I imagined she had. I wanted to be wanted. I wanted to be seen.

I still do.

The problem is that if being famous could give that to me, it already would have. Being seen at Living Foods, while not gliding on red carpets past clicking flashbulbs,

is still being seen. I could tell myself that it's not satisfying because I am not famous enough (thin enough,
beautiful enough, etc.). I could write myself a ten-
million-dollar check and spend the next five years devot-
ing myself to achieving more fame. I could spend the rest
of my life trying, or I could stop trying. But as soon as
I think of not trying, I feel like a doll with the stuffing
knocked out.

Trying gives me hope. Trying to be thin, trying to be
famous, trying to change. As long as I keep trying, there
is the possibility that someday I will make the mark, win
the race.

I tell this to my meditation teacher, Jeanne, who asks
me what I will win when I finally win the race.

"My father forever," I say, surprised at my answer.
"And then I will never be alone."

Fame and power were my father's gods. He was
moody and quiet, worked from five in the morning until
eleven at night. But when he talked about famous people, he came alive. He gestured with his hands, talked in
a lilting voice, wanted me to know that this was important, *they* were important. Our library was lined with
books about the Kennedys, the Rothschilds, the Wind-
sors. And movie stars. Cary Grant, Frank Sinatra, Judy
Garland. One night when I was twelve, he played Judy
Garland singing "Over the Rainbow" on the record of
The Wizard of Oz, followed by her rendition of the same
song thirty years later, at the Palace in London. As we
cuddled on the black and white paisley couch in the
basement, he spoke of the maturation of Judy Garland's

voice in hushed, reverent tones. I had him then—his attention, his love, his presence—and I didn't want to lose him. "Again, Daddy," I said. "Play the song again."

I don't remember deciding that I wanted to be one of the people whom he talked about in hushed, reverent tones. I don't remember deciding that if I was famous, I would be assured of his love and attention forever. Nor do I believe that the desire to be famous stems solely from the desire to have my father's love. But what I do believe is that I have an inherited image of myself as incapable and fat and dumb, and that I have used the desire to be thin and famous as antidotes to that image. It is the image that causes me pain, not the lack of fame. Until the image changes, nothing will make a difference. And when the image changes, fame, or the lack of it, will not matter.

Jeanne says, "We live our lives according to a tape made thirty years ago by people we wouldn't even ask directions from today."

I giggle at the image of standing in a gas station and asking my father or mother for directions to my life. I giggle because as absurd as it is, I've been following their directions for forty years. But if I stop, then it means that I have to let go of my parents as they live inside me. That sounds liberating, but I've been living with their company for so long, I'm not sure who I am without them.

Jeanne asks, "Who is this person that you spend most of your life trying not to be?"

I let myself into the pool of myself, beneath the trying, and when I do, I feel quiet and still. It doesn't feel bad.

I don't feel like I thought I would feel—clumsy and fat and dumb. I feel relieved, I feel calm, I feel whole. The silence is full, tinged with red and gold shimmers, like dust motes in the air.

Could this really be what I have been so afraid to feel? Thirty years of running from silence that is full and red and gold?

I take two jars of peanut butter, crunchy and smooth, and place them in the cart.

Last month I led a workshop in Seattle. During a visualization I asked people to walk up to a house covered with flowers that bore their name on a plaque in front. When they walked in the door, they faced a long hallway with three closed doors. Behind the first door was a room filled with their favorite foods, foods they craved or hardly allowed themselves to eat. When they entered this room they could do anything they wanted with the food—ignore it, eat it, taste it, touch it, take a bath in it. Then they walked to the second closed door. Behind it was something that nourished them—a person, an activity, an object, a situation. They saw themselves engaging with what was in the room, saw how they were nourished by whatever was there. When they walked to the door of the last room, they stood outside for a moment. They were told that this room contained their heart's desire, and when they opened the door, they were going to see what it was. Then they opened the door and spent as long as they liked with their heart's desire.

After the fantasy I asked people to speak about their experiences. One woman said that behind the door of her heart's desire was a feeling of wholeness that she had always wanted but had never felt. Another woman said that she hadn't yet found the work she wanted to do, but the room was filled with the feeling of doing it. I asked if anyone saw food or being thin in the room of their heart's desire. No one did. Then I asked if anyone saw a person in this room. No one did. Without exception, everyone in the room felt deeply satisfied by what they found in this room, whereas the experience of the other two rooms were described in terms of "lovely" and "sweet" or "don't care if I go back." Their heart's desire was not a thing, not a person, not something they could touch. It was a state of being, a response to a situation; it was already inside them.

I can't say this for sure, but I imagine that if I had done this fantasy five years ago, when the *New York Times* bestseller list was posted on my desk lamp, being famous would have had nothing to do with my heart's desire.

It still doesn't.

We think we already know what we want, what will make us happy. But most of those desires are based on trying to avoid, fix, or shore up old images of ourselves. We want to be thin because we have an identity of being fat and dumb, the kid that Ricky Gleason tortured in fifth grade, the girl who was sexually abused by her uncle, the child who was unwanted by her parents. And so we get thin, not because it feels good to be light, not because we enjoy eating particular foods, but to prevent ourselves from drowning in the thirty-year-old pain of being fat and dumb and unwanted. Then, since being thin does not change the image or make the pain go away, we gain back the weight so that we can pretend that when we lose it again, we will be happy. Or we decide that we need something else. A child, a lover, different work, more money, a toned body.

A woman in the workshop said that what she had wanted most as a child was for her mother to love her. She remembered taking her mother's gloves and sleeping with them next to her face. Remembered watching her mother get dressed in a pink silk blouse and thinking that she was the most beautiful woman in the world. She spoke of the longing and how it had twisted its way through her life, how she learned to hide it because she felt unwanted by her mother, how she learned to be embarrassed by it because her mother drank and made fun of her. She cut herself off from the integrity of her deepest desire—wanting to be loved—and layered herself with images of a girl her mother made fun of, didn't want. And she stayed that way. She was sixty-eight years old at the time of the workshop; her mother had been dead for twenty years.

We come into the world with our authenticity intact. Slowly, we realize that our parents can't see us (because they can't see themselves), don't know us (because they don't know themselves), and if we want their love, we must dress in a costume that pleases them. After years of wearing it, we think the costume is who we are, even when it gets tight and tattered. We get so attached to the costume that we refuse, no matter what the cost, to give it up; it is all we remember of ourselves. Our efforts to change usually consist of adding buttons or trim or rhinestones to the costume; the thought of removing it— letting go of our parents as they live in our bodies—is disorienting, even frightening.

Over the years I've made many improvements in my costume. But it still covers a girl who feels unwanted and unseen, which, paradoxically, is reassuring because it gives me something to do: I sparkle harder. I try to be beautiful, I try to be successful, I try to be famous, I try, I try, I try. And although my efforts actually achieve some wonderful things, things I really want, if I never take the costume off, my image of myself remains the same.

Was it fabulous to be on the bestseller list for even two weeks?

Absolutely.

It was a symbol that my work was reaching people, and it was the fruition of many years of work. It was many glorious things, but I didn't enjoy it because it didn't do what I wanted it most to do: change my experience of living in my body. The difference between how I felt and how I thought I would feel disappointed me so much that I was desperate to keep the book on the list, convinced that it wasn't *getting on*, it was *staying on*, that would make the difference.

My age-old belief is that if I stop trying, everything will fall apart and I won't get anything done. I will fall into the endless pit of eating chocolate and wearing muumuus and gaining five hundred pounds. My belief is that fat-and-dumb-and-ugly is always nipping at my heels, and if I stop trying, stop running, it will catch me, take me over. (This fear, as Jeanne points out, does not account for the fact that writing and teaching are two great passions of my life, and that I do them because they bring me joy, not because they bring me fame.)

We need some quinoa noodles, elbows, and rotelles. I wheel the cart around the corner, pick up three boxes of noodles, reach for a jar of Aunt Millie's Tomato Sauce with mushrooms and garlic. Put it next to the pasta.

Matt walks up behind me, drops a half gallon of apple juice into the cart. Three bottles of Calistoga, two packages of teriyaki tofu, a quart of Brown Cow yogurt.

"They don't have cherry cider," he says. "What else do we need?" He looks down at the cart, sees three boxes of quinoa noodles, two jars of peanut butter, a jar of tomato sauce and three bags of melted fruit. "You haven't gotten very far, honey. What have you been doing all this time?"

"Thinking about wearing muumuus and eating chocolate and what would happen if I stopped pushing myself."

No response.

I continue. "I act as if I don't believe there's a person with true passions beneath the pushing and trying. I need the fame to bolster what doesn't feel real."

"Would you mind if we talked about this when we got home?" Matt asks. "I find it hard to talk about Reality and Truth next to toilet paper and screaming babies. Get the rice and the popcorn, I'll get the zucchini. What else do we need?"

I take out the list from my pocket. "Salmon, lettuce, shiitake mushrooms, Napa cabbage."

He heads toward the vegetables. I take a few steps toward the bulk-food bins. Stop at the row of rice. Basmati rice, wild rice, brown rice, black rice. I rip off a plastic bag from the roll on the top shelf, scoop the basmati rice into the bag. Move to the popcorn. There's something so reassuring about hanging on to the image of myself as forever hungry and neurotic. I know how to be a child who wants, not a woman who has. Matt approaches with both arms full, a bag of zucchini falling on the floor. He bends down to pick it up, walks to the cart, drops the bags of food in.

"Remind me not to come here with you when you are in the middle of a chapter," he says.

I've spent twenty years in therapy and thirteen years of Buddhist practice trying to change, trying to convince myself that I am no longer unseen, unwanted, fat or ugly, and that the past is gone—be in the present, Geneen, get over yourself. I've probably spent more time analyzing the desire to be thin than Einstein spent developing the theory of relativity. I've spent years ashamed of, and then trying to talk myself out of, the desire to be famous by telling myself how superficial and shallow and unspiritual it is.

Therapy provided me with brilliant insights, and meditation provides me with a way to focus and concentrate my mind, but neither one has erased the image or helped me to stop wanting what I want.

Finally, it gets down to this: Take the costume off. Let myself know the part of me that feels forever fat and ugly, no matter what I look like or what I do. Focus on the reasons I want to hang on to the image rather than my need to get rid of it or pretend it's not there.

Years ago, when I realized that I was using food to express deep currents of feelings that I didn't know how to express any other way, I stopped dieting because I sensed that it had taken me as far as it could. I'd used it as a life raft to bring me to the other shore, and although I was on land now, I was still dragging the raft behind me.

I knew how to diet. I knew how to binge. I knew how to beat myself up for gaining weight and congratulate myself for losing weight. I didn't know how to be, eat, define myself without hanging on to the raft of dieting.

Fifteen years later, it is another round, deeper in the spiral. This time I am dragging the image of being fat and ugly behind me despite the fact that I am on the other shore.

I know how to be thin and believe I am fat. I know how to be successful and believe I am a failure. I don't know how to let myself alone. I don't act as if I trust the organic, luminous intelligence of the heart.

But this is what I *do* trust:

I trust the longing to be wanted, to be seen, to be loved.

The most painful thing about the woman in the workshop whose mother did not want her was not her mother's lack of love, but that in seeing herself the way her mother saw her, she cut herself off from her own love. Her longing to be seen by her mother was an expression of her need to have her own value reflected back to her.

We believe that because being wanted and being seen and being loved once depended on someone else, they still do. Because our experiences of wholeness were taken away by the reflections we received from other people, we believe we need those same reflections to retrieve that wholeness. So we keep finding goddesses to worship, keep hoping that more fame, a thinner body, more love will fill the hole, but since those things were not what caused the hole to begin with, they cannot possibly fill it now. When we open the door to the room of the heart's desire, there is no one to find but ourselves.

Wanting is the heart's way of saying, "Don't stop here, this isn't it." Wanting goes through a process of refinement, if you allow it. It goes from wanting shelter and warmth and enough to eat to wanting work that is fulfilling to wanting to be thin to wanting to be in love to wanting to be rich to wanting to be famous to wanting to be beautiful to wanting to be real to wanting to be free. But at every turn we have to stop, have to notice the pain, the dissatisfaction of getting what we want. We have to pay attention. We have to tell the truth. We have to understand that our need to see goddesses outside ourselves is an unwillingness to integrate and absorb all the fragmented, goddess pieces of ourselves.

When we clothe the heart's desire in the longing to be thin or to be famous or to be rich, we are doing the only thing that, as children, we could have done: We are forgetting who we are. Our journey now is not to stop wanting what we want, but to tell the truth about what happens when we get what we want, and to keep unlayering ourselves until we discover the connection between what we want and who we are.

I trust that the truth won't destroy me.

I trust that if we can allow ourselves to feel what we have spent our lives trying not to feel, it won't be horrible, it won't destroy us. I trust that our capacity to feel radiant and completely alive resides in our willingness to feel the very parts we've closed off.

I trust that I am not alone in my desire for the truth.

Support is available; there are people—teachers, friends—who are not afraid that they will be eaten by darkness, or who, conversely, are not afraid of joy, radiance, openness. It is important to find them.

I trust mistrust.

If we don't trust our desires, there are good reasons. Part of the work is to understand those reasons.

I trust the gentleness of the work, and that it is impossible to get rid of any part of myself.

The work is not to change who we are but rather to be who we are and to include every part of ourselves in our awareness. In other words, the work is not to be other than fat and ugly, but to understand why we cling to those images despite the existence of real passions, real motivations.

I trust that joy, radiance, satisfaction are possible as daily experiences.

What we thought we would get from being thin or being successful or being famous is still possible—it's just not in the places we've been looking. Or, as I heard in a meditation retreat recently: What we are looking for is who is looking.

Matt and I start walking to the checkout stand when I remember that we forgot to get nutmeg. "I'll be right back," I say. I walk to the row of spices, and a bottle of cinnamon reminds me of being with my mother the day before Thanksgiving a few years ago. We had been shopping for food all day long. Every time we got home, we remembered something else we hadn't bought. The fourth time, when we remembered we forgot the cinnamon, I had already changed into my nightgown.

"Oh, come on, sweetheart," my mother said, "just drive me down to Safeway. I'll run in. You won't even have to get out of the car."

"Okay, okay," I said. I put an old raincoat over my nightgown. The bottom layer of frills stuck out from the hem. Then I pulled on some rubber rain boots, a pair of sunglasses, and a baseball cap. I drove my mother to

Safeway and parked in front. "I'll wait right here," I said to her.

A guard walked over to me within five minutes. "Hey, lady," he said, "you have to move your car." I glanced at the ocean of cars in the half-acre parking lot, their windshields glinting like the crests of waves.

"But I'm waiting for my mother, and it's a madhouse in there. She'll never find me when she comes out."

"Sorry, lady," he said. "Fire regulations."

I glared at him and then drove to the other side of the lot. She'll never find me, I thought. I have to go find her.

My mother was nowhere to be seen. I used our method of finding each other in department stores: shouting each other's names. "Mom! Where are you?"

"Here I am. Over here," she shouted back.

She was next in line at the far checkout stand. I walked over to her, everyone now staring at our rude display of behavior. "I'm to the right when you walk out of the store, ten rows back. I'll wait for you in the car."

"Hey," the checkout woman said. "Hey, don't I know you from someplace? You look familiar."

"No," I said, "I don't know you. You must be mistaken."

"I could swear I've seen you before. I know you, I just know I know you."

I started to walk away. My mother grabbed the sleeve of my coat, pulled me back. "You know her because she's a *star*. You've probably seen her on many television shows, but just last week she was on *Oprah*. She is a star."

"Oh, yeah! Oh, wow! That's it! I saw you on *Oprah*. I actually ran out and bought your book. It's great, it's really great."

My mother smiled a wide, proud smile. Then she remembered that her alcoholic and drug-addicted years were described in the book. "By the way," she added, "I'm not really her mother."

We waltzed out of the store, arm in arm. My non-mother in her high heels and high cheekbones and me in my nightgown and rubber boots.

Chapter Three

▪

PARALLEL LIVES, PART 1: LOSING MY HAIR

▪

Women in my workshops say, "If someone loves me when I am fat, I know they truly love me. But if anyone comments that I look good because I lost weight, I wonder if they thought I looked terrible before. I want to be loved for who I am, not for being thin or looking good."

I wonder what that means, being loved for who you are. I know it doesn't mean physical appearance — weight, skin, clothes, hair. It means, I think, the qualities that cannot be weighed or measured. The texture of the soul.

I am wondering why, if all of us want to be loved for who we are, we spend so much energy trying to be someone else, trying to change the way we look, act, feel, think.

I am wondering who we think we are beneath the trying, and what would happen if we stopped trying. If all the ways we identify ourselves were suddenly taken away, if we couldn't work, couldn't exercise, couldn't make love, couldn't mother, couldn't use our faces, our bodies, our personalities, to pull us through. Then would we be who we really are?

I am thinking about this because my eyebrows and eyelashes are gone, my hair is falling out in fistfuls, and without the things I use to present myself to the world, I'm getting confused about who I am.

I was looking at pictures recently from our Caribbean vacation. In one picture Matt and I are on a beach, arms flung casually around each other's shoulders. The man we recruited to take the picture, a wiry, copper-haired fellow who we later discovered was a proctologist from Chicago, focused on my face and the palm tree in the background. Half of Matt's nose, eyes, and mouth are cut off. But my eyebrows are there, curved like seashells, arching demurely. The day the picture was taken I drank a virgin piña colada that tasted like coconut ice from La Guli's. Matt and I took a walk on a black sand beach, and he found a large conch shell the color of a ballerina's satin slippers. We went snorkeling and saw a baby turtle. My mask leaked water, and the fin on my right foot kept scraping my toe. I didn't spend one minute noticing or appreciating my eyebrows.

Now they are gone, along with my eyelashes and most of my hair.

I do not have cancer. I am not dying.

I have vitamin A poisoning, which I got because my doctor and I (the same doctor who put me on the Candida diet and whose office and counsel I have now abandoned) had a serious miscommunication. Instead of taking four drops a day, I took four droppers—the difference between twenty thousand units and four hundred thousand units. Since vitamin A is stored in the liver and is not washed out of the body in urine, it is an especially toxic vitamin to misuse; the symptoms will take six months to disappear. In the meantime a new plague develops every week. Bone and joint pain, weeping rashes, migraine headaches, bright orange skin. Every inch of my body itches and burns, but nothing compares to losing my hair.

I didn't have big hair to begin with, something which has plagued me since I was seven. Before I learned to blame my misfortunes on my fat, I blamed them on my hair. In fourth grade I was convinced that Mindy Goldfarb got the role of Anna in *The King and I* (and I the role of her understudy) because she had naturally curly hair that fell in thick banana curls on her shoulders. I had fine, thin hair that wouldn't curl or stay in a barrette for longer than ten minutes.

Every time, through all the years, my mother and I are on an escalator in a department store (and believe me, this is a statistically significant number of times), she notices a woman riding in the opposite direction, someone with hair as thick as Niagara Falls (usually red, usually long), someone who looks as if she needs a lasso to hold her hair in a ponytail. I am usually in the middle of a sentence when my mother grabs my arm, uses her nose to point to the cloud of red, and says, "What a head of hair! Can you believe that head of hair? In my next life, please God, I am going to have thick hair." Sometimes, but not always, this sentence is followed by: "Of all the things you could have gotten from me, you had to get my hair." She sighs and makes a clucking sound with her tongue as the big red hair glides (ungratefully, we are certain) to home furnishings.

In our family, hair was a source of speculation and eccentric activities. My father started losing his hair when he was thirty and decided to wear a toupee—"like Frank Sinatra," he said, "blue-eyed and handsome." My mother wore hairpieces and switches—long braids twisted around French knots to make it look as if she had armloads of hair. During our frequent hair discussions, my mother would teach me what was appropriate in the hirsute world: Women over twenty-five should not wear hair down to their waists; thin hair should always be cut short; women over forty should not wear shoulder-length hair.

When I was six, my mother cut my bangs with nail scissors and made a diagonal swath up my forehead. The next day she sent me to Mary's Beauty Salon on Twenty-first Avenue for a cut and a perm. Mary, who had a large mole on her right cheek with a tuft of hair sprouting from it, set my hair in hard pink rollers, doused it with permanent solution, and waited for a miracle. It didn't happen. Except for a minor wave here or there, my hair refused to curl.

My days of glory arrived when girls began ironing their hair, setting it on soup can rollers, doing anything to make it look like the hair I was born with. Alas, with the arrival of the seventies, thick, bouncy hair made a comeback, and has been coming back ever since.

Ten years ago, I found Richard Johnson (an artist, I called him, a Picasso with scissors), who created magic with my hair. It looked swingy, shiny and, from certain angles (the back, the right side) even thick. I vowed my allegiance to him forever. I drove from Santa Cruz to San Francisco, a seventy-five-mile drive, every six weeks for five years. When he became an alcoholic, a drug addict, a compulsive liar, when he didn't show up for appointments, when he promised that he would cut my hair for a book tour, that I could come to his house and call him on the day of the appointment for directions, when he kept his phone off the hook that whole day while I called him every five minutes from a gas station in Palo Alto, waiting for him to keep his promise, certain he wouldn't betray me, I, like any woman who loves haircuts too much, stayed faithful, wishing and hoping he would change. Instead, he checked himself into a residential program for substance abuse and moved to Ashland, Oregon.

At first I thought that four hundred miles was too far to go for a haircut. Then I decided that it all depends on your point of view, and since distance is subjective, and since I believed that getting a good haircut was tantamount to healthy self-esteem, four hundred miles became a minor hurdle. I managed two-hour stopovers on my way to teach workshops in Portland, Seattle, Anchorage. Richard picked me up at the airport, drove me to the salon where he was working, gave me the haircut I yearned for, then drove me back to the plane. Sara and I made weekend adventures out of trips to Ashland. As soon as we got on Highway 5, we'd put the Supremes on the tape player, open the windows, and belt out "Baby Love" and "I Hear a Symphony" at the top of our lungs. We went to the Shakespeare festival, saw *Macbeth*, *Romeo and Juliet*, slept in ratty motel rooms. And most important, we got our swingy, bouncy haircuts. Then my frequent-flyer miles ran out, and after a few terrible haircuts from a few terrible hairdressers, I found an artist closer to home.

Although I could have gotten the award for "Woman Willing to Travel Farthest for a Haircut," the concept of defining oneself by appearance is not an alien one. Richard told me that when he was working for a well-known salon, a woman sued his boss for emotional trauma. She said that her hair looked like someone put a bowl over it and cut with their eyes closed, and that she spent four days crying and two weeks hiding in the house. The judge awarded her enough money for three hats.

Even Matt, my model of sanity and balance, got a haircut once from someone who didn't know how to cut his woolly hair, and when his head looked square like a box instead of round like a head, he complained for weeks. Once during that time I saw him looking in the mirror and trying to stretch his hair.

Most of us seem to believe, no matter what we say, that who we are is what we look like, and until something drastic happens, something about which we have no choice, we don't question that belief.

I had a boss once. His name was Phillip Packer, a high-powered executive who was also a triathlete, a husband, a father of two young children. He was a man with money, a man with a future, a man who knew who he was. After his yearly physical he was diagnosed with inoperable cancer. Within three months he was bedridden. His running shoes hung by their laces on his closet door; the keys to his red Mercedes convertible lay on a shelf in his dresser. His body, which he had built and toned and perfected for ten years became atrophied from lack of use. He couldn't pick up his children, couldn't make love with his wife, couldn't run his company, or take pleasure in his million-dollar house with the paintings he'd collected from Europe. His life became very simple (could he hear the birds in the morning? could he sit in the garden today? were the irises in bloom? could he read his children a story?), and as I sat with him in his sickroom, beside an oxygen tank and trays of medication, I was astonished to realize that I envied him.

I was sad, of course, that he was dying. I was horrified by how quickly it was happening, but there was a spaciousness about him, something peaceful and transparent about his presence. It was as if he had been living in one cramped, airless room of a mansion before his illness, and now he'd opened the doors to all the rooms. He could relax. There was no big thing to prove or do or look like anymore. No prize, no victory.

I was thirty years old, my first book was about to be published, and I was embroidering my dreams with the resplendent life that would soon be mine. As I watched

Phillip's physical body deteriorate and his openness expand, I decided that after I got famous, I would think of a way to feel peaceful and spacious without having to be sick, lose everything, and die.

"Shave it," I say to Elizabeth, my San Francisco stylist. "I can't stand to see it coming out in bunches, can't stand to see the blanket of hair on my pillow every morning. Just take an electric shaver and buzz it off."

"I don't think you are ready for that," she says. "It's a huge change. You don't need to be so drastic. I can cut your hair shorter and then, in a month, if you still want to shave it, we will."

I agree to a short haircut. She parts it in the middle instead of at the side, cuts it so that the bald spots don't show as much. From the back I don't look as if I am losing my hair. But in front I can see the pale curve of my scalp, bare as the moon in August.

It took me awhile to realize my hair was falling out. I was too itchy to think, feel, care about anything. I wanted to jump out of my skin, throw myself against a wall to stop the stinging, the burning. I tried pain medications, breathing into the sensations, asking myself what itching actually felt like. Was it on the surface of the skin or just below the surface? What color was it? What shape? The meditation helped for a while, an hour, maybe two. Then I would forget to breathe, start itching again, and feel terribly sorry for myself.

Then the itchiness began to subside, and with it the

nosebleeds, the headaches, the rashes. But while brushing my teeth one morning, I noticed that my face looked pale. Besides the dark brown baseball-sized blotches on my cheeks, also a result of the vitamin A, there was a monochromatic line from my eyes to my hair, and then I realized my eyebrows had fallen out. The fistfuls of hair on the pillow meant my hair was falling out. I stood at the sink and wept.

It's the nakedness that gets to me. The feeling of being exposed, of having nothing to hide behind. I used to be able to do my hair, put on some makeup, and look different than I felt. I could "put on my face," as my mother says. Now there is no way to feel attractive. I look like one of those old ladies in Miami Beach, the ones whose husbands have died, the ones who show up at Wolfie's Delicatessen wearing pink pearls and mink stoles with the heads and claws attached. From the neck down they look imposing. But they wear their vulnerability like a reluctant crown, shining through wispy hair.

I wander from room to room, stand at the kitchen window, stare at the gray cat curled up on a paisley wing chair in the next-door neighbor's apartment. I can see the neighbor's long legs when I stand at the sink. And her thick, honey-colored hair. Thousands of women, one in nine this year, will be diagnosed with breast cancer, undergo chemotherapy, and lose their hair. I weep for them as I chop a tomato, reach for a carrot. How will they cope, I wonder, with losing their hair *and* the necessity to make choices on which their lives depend? With losing their hair *and* losing a breast, two breasts? Matt tells me that when Lou Ann, his first wife, lost her hair from the chemotherapy she received for ovarian cancer, he went with her to cancer-support groups where everyone had lost their hair. At first, he says, it was a big deal. Then it was "So what? We lost our hair, it's only hair."

It's only hair, I tell myself over and over, like a mantra, like a song: "It's only hair, they're only eyebrows. My face is not me." I don't believe myself. It's not only hair, they're not only eyebrows. My face *is* me. I didn't know that before, but I know it now. If I thought meditating daily for thirteen years had helped me detach from temporal phenomena, I was wrong.

My friend Moo tells me about the day she cut her hair, when she was thirty-three (the year Jesus was crucified, she emphasizes, a very significant time in anyone's life). She went to the beach with a friend, they brought their drums and scissors, and after chanting to Ceres, the underwater goddess, the one with seaweed and snakes writhing from her hair (isn't that Medusa? I ask her. Aren't you confusing the goddess of hair with the one who turned everyone to stone?), and they cut, chanted, drummed. Hair is a big deal, she tells me. Look at cornrows, look at dreadlocks. It's the way people express who they are, their heritage, their significance in the world. But, I ask her, does it follow that if you lose your hair, you lose your significance? Of course not, she answers, don't be silly. Being silly, I assure her, is the furthest thing from my mind.

I slog through the day as if underwater. I watch healthy people, people with energy, people with eyebrows, move quickly through crowds, up a flight of steps. They seem like strangers from another planet, aliens who don't have to disperse their energy in small parcels.

I keep asking Matt if he is repulsed by the bald spots, the lack of eyebrows, eyelashes, and he keeps telling me he loves me no matter what. "It's a look," he says, "like those pierced eyebrows, and neon mohawks we see on Telegraph Avenue. You fit right in."

I giggle and say, "Really? You really still love me? You really aren't sickened by the way I look?"

"Honey," he says, "it doesn't matter to me, it really doesn't."

I love you no matter what. The no-matter-what part is the part that catches in my throat.

"If I killed someone, you wouldn't love me," I tell him, "so it's not true that you love me no matter what."

He sighs. "You wouldn't kill anyone, Geneenie, you really wouldn't. You wouldn't do anything that betrays the essence of you. That's what I am talking about. That's why I can say the no-matter-what part."

Easy for him to say—he trusts "the essence." I don't even know what the essence is or who he sees; I only know that this is not the way my life is supposed to look. Losing my hair is not part of the plan. I know how things are supposed to unfold. If I make the right decisions, have the right body, the right hair, make a success of myself, then life will go smoothly and I will be loved.

The only "no matter what" I know is that no matter what happens to convince me differently, I still believe in this parallel life. I still place inordinate emphasis, living-and-dying emphasis, on how I look and what I do, on what I produce and what I achieve, on how I perform and what I say or do or look like on a given day. Each moment rests on the next, waits breathlessly to see if I deserve the next.

I catch myself living in my parallel world during a variety of activities: before I go to sleep at night; when I daydream; after I finish a book and before it gets published; if I read *Vogue* or *People*; and when I try on clothes. I see Matt and me getting dressed up and going to the opera (he hates opera), the ballet (he doesn't like that, either) or some other place in the city (I don't like the city) where we need clothes like the ones I am trying on. In this parallel world, people are thin, have big hair, and spend their lives sweeping into places, swirling in black taffeta dresses with glittering eyes. In this world, being beautiful means something and being famous makes people happy and being thin opens the golden door of the universe.

As a child I believed in a world where appearance counted because beauty and money and fame were the altars at which everyone I knew worshiped, and because appearance was the only thing I could actually control. The twin goals of being thin and being famous gave me something to work toward: the belief that if I achieved them, my mother would love me. At the same time they gave me a way out of my broken family.

As an adult I have been thin for fifteen years, been famous at Living Foods grocery store and within a small sector of the population (those who read my books), and I am still waiting to be thin and famous. To live in the promised world. I didn't think I was waiting, but losing my hair convinces me differently.

I feel the despair of someone who has lost her chance. People with bald heads are not beautiful, do not sweep into rooms, do not wear black taffeta dresses. I can no longer pretend that another life is waiting around the corner (no matter that I love my husband, my work, my community, no matter that this life is my life, the one I created, the one I want), I am still waiting for the love, the glory, the prize. I am still trying to be the girl my mother can love.

Last week I picked up a copy of *Vogue*, turned to the last page first. A page of glittering diamond bracelets. I found myself musing about wearing the thick one, the one studded with emeralds. In my other life, the one where I sweep into rooms wearing ballgowns, I look ravishing in the emerald and diamond cuff. Halfway into a scintillating conversation with a famous artist, I reminded myself that in my present world I am bald. Also, I spent most of the day in my writing outfit—a faded sky blue jumpsuit that is twelve years old with blotches of red ink, ragged sleeves, and legs that are five inches above my ankles.

Next, I turned to an article about supermodels. I spent years waiting to grow up so that I could look like a model, convinced that growing up meant growing out of my body and into a new one. When I was sixteen, I finally realized that these legs weren't getting any longer, and this hair wasn't getting any bigger. I was never going to look like Veronica in the Archie comics. It was a shock.

I'm not alone. Forty thousand girls apply to be models every year. Four of them make it. The problem is that having a five-feet-ten, hundred-and-twenty-pound body is the exception, not the rule. One hundredth of one percent of women who apply have the right body. This does not include the ones who don't apply but wish they could. The ones who are sitting home waiting to grow taller, wanting to slice off pieces of their thighs, their arms, so that they can look like a waif. This does not include the average American woman, who is five-feet-three, weighs a hundred and forty pounds, and is a size fourteen.

In the *Vogue* article, the supermodels talked about their flaws. Christy Turlington, referred to as "the most beautiful woman in the world," said, "I know how to make every part of my body appear different than it actually is. I can make my eyes and my lips appear bigger by putting my chin down. I can make my hips appear smaller. I can make my chest appear bigger. You can manipulate everything for photography."

Which means even she doesn't look like herself. I remember a fourteen-year-old girl on the *Jenny Jones* show, an anorexic who weighed sixty pounds. She wanted to look like Claudia Schiffer, but what she was seeing in the magazines wasn't really Claudia Schiffer. It was a manipulated image, a fake.

How can we compete with images? Is it more important to look like a model who chain-smokes, bites her nails, and lives on pasta without sauce than to look like ourselves? What would we, as women, look like, feel like, live like, if we gathered the energy we spend on trying to make our hips appear smaller, our lips appear bigger, and spent it on truth telling, on learning about, and then becoming, who we actually are?

Most of us will never have lives like the people we read about in magazines, see on movie screens, or watch on television. At the end of the movie we still have to inhabit our own lives. And if we spend those lives trying to have someone else's life, we will never know who we actually are.

My friend Shirley lost eighty pounds seven years ago, and has kept it off by eating a low-fat diet and exercising six days a week "no matter what." Last month she fell down a flight of steps and fractured her leg in three places. The doctor says she won't be able to exercise for three months, and Shirley is terrified. "What am I going to do?" she asks. "I need to be active. I'm not the kind of person who can sit around all day. I'm going to lose my mind. And I'm going to gain weight. That's the worst part. Having a broken leg is bad, but gaining weight is worse." If she can't run three miles a day, if she gains fifteen pounds, if her main way of coping with the world— through constant activity—is taken from her, who is she?

At some point we have to reckon with ourselves; we will never feel loved for who we are until we discover who we are. We have to decide in which parts of ourselves to invest meaning. Are we our faces? Our bodies? Our relationships? Our work?

Even with a life of perfect health and big hair, we will still get wrinkled and old. The many ways (body, career, parenting, partnering) in which we identify ourselves will change, and we will be left with the task of finding the restorative thread of ourselves—our essence—in our day-to-day lives.

I decide to go to Tassajara, a Zen mountain-retreat center in Carmel Valley. No one will know me there, and the monks are bald. I can study the creases in their scalps, notice how necks look when there is no hair carpeting them. I can meditate, try to get some perspective on the situation, remind myself that I am not dying, it's only hair. In the baths I see a woman who has lost both breasts, has one arm that is three times the size of the other. I watch as she maneuvers out of her wheelchair and slides into the hot water. We are the only ones in the tub. A bluejay caws, and the woman asks my name. What I really want to answer is, "My name is Geneen and I've been sick for three years and I am losing my hair, but I have both my breasts and I am not in a wheelchair, so will you tell me how you make sense of your life?" Instead, we talk about how many years each of us has been coming to Tassajara, about living in Berkeley, about our work—she is celebrating her seventieth birthday; her new book will be released in the fall.

In the baths the next morning, I gather my courage and ask her when she lost her breasts, why she's in a wheelchair. She tells me about having polio fifty years ago, about having breast cancer thirty years ago, about the radiation that enlarged her arm, the post-polio syndrome that has put her in a wheelchair. I tell her about being diagnosed with chronic fatigue syndrome, Candida, vitamin A poisoning.

"But it's losing my hair that has sent me over the edge," I say, "and I am stuck in the grief of it. I feel silly for caring so much about my hair. I'm not in a wheelchair, I'm not dying."

She is looking at me with so much compassion that it makes me cry. "Will you tell me how you manage so many physical losses?" I ask.

"You can't compare one sickness with another. I don't think about being in a wheelchair. I don't let it stop me from living my life. I'm not self-conscious about having no breasts.

"But last week I got an awful haircut, and when I look in the mirror, my hair bothers me terribly. When I don't like my hair, I don't like the way I look, and that is what makes me self-conscious."

I stare at her, dumbfounded, then begin to laugh. I realize I am hearing fifty years' worth of coming to terms with illness, and a week's worth of irritation about her hair, but still, the idea that her hair bothers her releases me from my shame and loneliness.

I spend the week writing, taking naps, eating warm, crusty homemade bread with fruit soups. I read Reynolds Price's book *A Whole New Life*. Price writes that after an appallingly painful and life-altering battle with cancer, after becoming a paraplegic, after years of howling and suffering, when he compares his present life to his past, he'd "have to say that, despite an enjoyable fifty-year start, these recent years since full catastrophe have gone still better."

Better. He says his life is better now than it was when he could walk, run, go the bathroom without Olympic maneuvers. He says, "I've yet to watch another life that seems to have brought more pleasure to its owner than mine has to me." If his life is better now, when he can't live alone, when his legs are limp, dead fish hanging from his torso, when he is in constant pain, it is because he has taken the pain and traveled with it, taken the suffering and planted it in the seething, fertile soil of his consciousness, where patience grows from endless hours of waiting and love pushes through. Where the sheer pleasure of friendship and work and eros are enough—if you are willing to be melted and forged by the pain. If you are not attached to matching your life with the way you think life needs to be. If you accept yourself the way you are.

This much I know from losing my hair: My face doesn't look like me, and yet the part of me that is most me has not changed. As long as I keep hanging on and trying to go back to the old me, as long as I think I know what I am supposed to have, look like, and be, as long as I keep rejecting what I have now in favor of a fantasy of what I think will make me happy, I will be frustrated and in pain.

We can accept the way we are or reject it. Rejection takes many forms: shame; an intense focus on self-improvement; the belief that if we left ourselves alone, we would never work, we would never exercise, we would wear pink rollers and watch soap operas and eat chocolate all day long. Rejection can feel like determination, willpower, relentlessness to change. Fantasizing about a parallel life is a rejection of ourselves, our present lives.

Acceptance is believing that we want to know the truth, and that there is a part of us, our "essence," that recognizes truth, that clings to truth. Essence is the part that cannot be weighed or measured. It's the you that remains when your body has cancer and you can't lift your children, when you break a leg and can't exercise every day, when you overdose on vitamin A and lose your hair. When everything you thought you were disappears, there is still something that remains. A being-ness, an is-ness, a presence. And it is that something (and the recognition of it) that brings peace, strength, fulfillment, happiness.

I observe that I am pulled between a basic trust of myself and a basic fear. Between letting myself alone and believing that if I don't shove myself, I will never move.

Since I lost my hair, I have been pushing myself, punishing myself, blaming myself. I have told myself that anyone with brains can tell the difference between a drop and a dropper. I have told myself that the real me is mean-spirited and fat, and that she *deserves* to lose her hair, to flail in a pool of illness and bad luck for the next twenty lifetimes. That basic rejection of myself, the cruelty with which I treat myself, glues my thoughts together, makes it impossible to feel anything but self-loathing. The distance between who I think I need to look like and the "real me" is so wide that the only thing I can do is drive myself harder and harder, until one day I give up and run the other way.

Another alternative is to stop running. It is to actually ask myself what is real here:

Is it true that I am stupid?

How stupid do I think I am?

And what about the selfish and mean-spirited and fat part? Am I really fat? Mean-spirited? If I believe those things, why do I believe them?

What did I want that I could never have, which made me feel like an endless pit of need?

What do I imagine would happen if I responded to pain with softness and vulnerability instead of self-recriminations about how I am not doing it right?

My task right now is not necessarily to answer these questions, but to understand that the way I respond to loss and pain doesn't help them go away; it creates more pain.

I look carefully at the naked heads of the Tassajara monks. I decide that I like the folds in bare scalps, that I prefer round heads to pointy heads, that if much more of my hair falls out, I will shave my head and, for the first time in my adult life, see the shape of my scalp, run the palm of my hand on the crown of my head, feel the softness, the smoothness, bare pink skin touching bare pink skin.

When I notice myself believing that only people with hair (with thin bodies, who work at politically and spiritually correct work for little or no money and if not that, then they are as famous and rich as Julia Roberts) deserve kindness, I remind myself that that voice is not my friend, is not true, is not real. This takes a lot of reminding. It takes a long time.

But slowly, over the next few months, I find myself relaxing into the hair loss, touching the bald spots gently. I begin to have confidence that if my hair never grows back, if I am sick for the next forty years the way I have been for the past three years, I will carve a new life for myself. I will stop trying to be who I was with hair and a healthy body. I will become who I am, with no eyebrows, no eyelashes, no hair, a quarter of the energy. My face *was* me—the me I was when I looked like I used to look. My face is still me—me without hair, with dark brown blotches, with orange skin. My life is still mine.

But it is a different life, I am not the same me as I was before.

The truth of losing my hair is that it evokes memories of never being good enough, of feeling awkward and dumb and ugly. The truth of losing my hair is that nothing has happened except that I've lost my hair. I still have my work, my friends, my cat, my life, myself. Nothing has changed except that I can no longer pretend I am about to have one of those lives that only people with big hair deserve.

A few weeks ago Matt suggested that I call my friend Patty, who makes clothes, hats, jewelry. We visited her apartment, where we bought two flowered hats for the days I don't want to go to the grocery store bald. One of the hats is dark burgundy velvet with a moss green silk peony pinned to the front. The effect is luscious, and I am glad to have something so beautiful and soft for my head, which has been the recipient, since the vitamin A fiasco, of so much self-inflicted harshness.

Patty serves us peach crumble with vanilla bean ice cream, and as I sit there, on her blue and white seersucker couch tasting the tang of peach, the sweet flash of brown sugar, I realize it doesn't get any better than this: sitting on a seersucker couch in the middle of Tuesday in the middle of my life, with no desire to be anywhere or anyone else.

A year has passed.

During the past six months my hair has grown back,

along with my eyebrows and eyelashes. Due to a few circumstances—working with a brilliant doctor, meeting weekly with a spiritual teacher, and being willing to work with myself—I am well again. I am more than well; I feel vital and resilient, better than I have in twenty years.

People say to me, "You passed through a dark night of the soul, and from that darkness healing came," but it's not that simple. While it is true that losing my hair was the nadir of three years of progressive illness, and while dark nights are always followed by dawns, it is not necessarily true that healing follows pain or that health follows illness or that safety follows terror.

The outcome of a challenging or disappointing or horrifying situation depends on how you use it.

Losing my hair made it impossible for me to lie. I'd spent my life believing that if I showed my vulnerability, if I showed anyone they had the power to hurt me, I would be destroyed. This belief was, like all beliefs, composed of layers. Yes, I'd let Matt into my life, and yes, I'd written personal, revealing books, and yes, I'd had close friends with whom I'd been intimate. But I still held a core belief that it was better to hide, that it was, in fact, necessary to hide parts of myself. This belief was attached to an image of myself as a cowering child who learned that who she was, her barest truth, was wrong and shameful, and that revealing herself gave people more ammunition with which to hurt her. The only way to keep safe and maintain control, therefore, was to layer myself with false gaiety and indifference to being hurt.

Anyone who would travel four hundred miles for a

haircut had to believe that something very important rested on her ability to look good. That if she didn't look as good as it was possible to look, something terrible would happen. Anyone who would travel four hundred miles for a haircut had to be certain that her survival depended on creating distraction from whom she believed herself to be.

Without hair I felt stripped and naked and raw, with no possibility of being anything or anyone else. It was as if everything I had been covering up for forty years came hurtling to the surface. When you believe, as I did, that it is impossible to be loved for who you really are, and if you reveal yourself, you will be destroyed, losing your main mask—your physical appearance—is terrifying.

While I am well aware that anyone who loses her hair usually goes through a period of despair, that is not the point. The point is what these kinds of losses (broken legs, illnesses, accidents, sudden losses of any kind) evoke in us. The point is being given the chance to see parts of ourselves that we would never choose to see voluntarily. They are there, in us, these self-images, these core beliefs, operating at an unconscious level all the time, keeping us from knowing ourselves, from being in the present, from knowing ourselves to *be* presence. The poet Audre Lorde said that no pain is ever wasted if we learn from it. If we use the situations that are given to us as chances to see the secrets we are keeping from ourselves, each one of us can be a Reynolds Price.

It depends on what we think we are alive to do. If life is about acquiring, if it's about matching our lives to our dream lives, we will not learn from our losses; we will be no different at the end of a crisis than at the beginning of it. We will rail against the gods and declare ourselves the unlucky victims of unlucky circumstance. If life is about inquiring into the ways we keep ourselves from being awake and open and true, then no pain will ever be wasted. Then broken egg shells will be used as compost for Blue Moon roses.

I wish I could say that now, a year later, with a full head of hair, I no longer spend even a moment as that cowering, dumb child, but it's not true. If I lost my hair again, I would still go through a period of depression and terror, and I would probably believe myself to be unlovable, but after the initial resistance and bout of self-pity, I would enter the pain again, and another layer of the old self-image would be shed.

Most women will never lose their hair. Most people will never get cancer and become paraplegics. But everyone has disappointments and illnesses that evoke deep-seated, unconscious self-images. We know we are in the grip of one of these images when we respond to a situation with feelings of being completely bad, unworthy, unlovable, ugly, empty. When we feel victimized, when we swing from obsessing about what the other person did wrong to being unable to remember anything kind or decent about ourselves, an old image is being reactivated, and this image is keeping us from knowing the fullness of who we are.

It doesn't matter why something happens. Why you got cancer or why you lost your hair or why you got into a car accident. What matters is what you do with it. What matters is how you use it. What matters is getting your life back. And since all you have to work with is who you are and what you're given, you might as well use them. There is nothing else to do except punish yourself or whine or feel like a victim.

We are more than our hair, our faces, our bodies, our relationships. But we will never know that until we understand the images that keep us from remembering ourselves. When they are recognized, they dissolve. And when they dissolve, we become that much freer to be the vastness of who we are.

There is no other prize. Of that I am confident.

Chapter Four

■

WHEN SOMEONE
BELIEVES IN YOU

■

It is September of 1989 and I am walking up Madison Avenue to Peg's apartment building. As I turn the corner on Ninety-sixth Street, the beefy smells of Jackson Hole, the hamburger joint on the corner, make me start thinking about, and then craving, a medium-rare burger with pickles, mayonnaise, mustard, lettuce, and tomatoes on a sesame seed bun. It's been a long time since I've eaten meat, but hamburgers were always my favorite. I felt so American when I ate them. As if I belonged.

I ring Peg's doorbell, 21G. I wait a long time, hear a cane tapping on the floor, tap, walk, tap, tap walk tap, the sound of the chains being pulled open, keys turning in their locks, and there she is, in a long black cotton skirt and a brown-and-white-striped blouse. Chunky jewelry around her neck, on her ears. She looks thinner than ever, as if the earth is barely holding on to her. The circles around her eyes are darker than the last time I saw her, six months ago, and there is a weariness about her shoulders, her eyes.

She reaches out her hand. "Well, hello, my dear," she says.

I take her hand, kiss her cheek. "Hi, Peg. I've missed you. I'm glad you could have dinner with me tonight."

"Come in for a moment while I get my purse."

As soon as I walk into her living room, I remember why I don't like this room. The frills on the Laura Ashley pink-striped curtains do nothing to change the feeling I have here: there is a vortex in the center of this room that sucks the light out of the plants, flowers, animals, relationships. It's a dark and dank space, and the pack of cigarettes on the table is the only thing that looks as if it belongs. I tell myself that her house in East Quogue must be different, brighter. Peg gardens there, she cooks there.

"Shall we go to Marybeth's Kitchen?" Peg asks as she slings her small black purse around one shoulder and begins tapping her way to the door with the other arm.

"Where else?" I answer. I walk in back of her, notice that her purse is hitting her hip, ask if I can carry it.

"No," she says firmly, "I am not an invalid."

We stand at the corner waiting for the light to change. It is September and balmy; I am in New York for the Jewish holidays. When the green light flashes, we begin walking slowly to the other side of Madison, which suddenly seems like a continent away. It takes us a green light and part of a red light to get across. "It's amazing," Peg says, "how even the damn taxi drivers are patient when you have a cane."

The host seats us at a corner table. Peg rests her cane

on the wall behind me. Since she fell on a bus and cracked her hip, then got fired from Bobbs-Merrill, she has felt useless and bored. I encourage her to apply for jobs at other publishing companies, but she says she is too old. The positions are being filled with twenty-year-olds. (They want whippersnappers in there, Geneen, and I don't fit the description. You are the original whipper-snapper, I say, and a fabulous editor. The best.)

I am incensed that she can't get a job. I have tried getting her a job at my new publishing company. They say they will hire her on a freelance basis, but she has been working every day for forty years and wants a full-time job. I want her to have stacks of manuscripts by her bed, something around which to wrap that fire in her mind.

Peg orders salmon with garlic aioli. I order a Caesar salad and vegetable linguine. She is telling me about her friend Sam, who writes fairy tales for children. Her neck-lace of hexagonal crystal beads is throwing a rainbow on the stuccoed wall. As she sits there, hands gesturing, I love her more than I have ever loved anyone, ever. She remembers everything I tell her: my friends' names, how much my cat Blanche weighs, the fight my father and I had last week.

It is beginning to get dark, and a waiter wearing a bo-lero jacket comes around to light three small candles at our table. Her cane keeps crashing to the floor. I keep picking it up, leaning it at an angle, turning around to see her face.

"Peg?"

"Yes?"

"Peg, is there anything that I can do for you, anything at all?"

"Keep writing, Geneen. Listen to Auntie Peg."

"No, I mean, *for you*. What can I do *for you* . . ."

"You're already doing it. You're here, talking to me, being with me, you keep sending me your manuscripts to work on. I need to work."

"But what about the pain, Peg?"

"Now listen, don't start talking to me like I'm in one of your workshops. My pain is my own business. I'm in therapy, have been for a million years, and I'm doing the best I can."

I take a deep breath, ask myself if I have the courage to say what I see, what I believe. Tell myself there is nothing to lose, so I might as well speak up. "The way you drink, and the way you smoke, gives me the feeling that you want to die."

"Oh, hogwash. Who said anything about dying?"

"I did. You go at it with such a vengeance. Why won't you talk about it?"

"Plenty of people drink and smoke without wanting to die. Stop fancying that grandiose intuition of yours. I appreciate the concern, but please—leave your analyses for your books. I just want your company."

I sigh. I had a feeling I wasn't going to get anywhere with this conversation, but I'm still glad I brought it up. "I just want you to know that I love you and I would do anything for you."

"And you are loved as well."

I pick up a cornbread stick, begin spreading it with

strawberry butter. "We've come a long way since that first meeting eight years ago . . ." I say. "Did I ever tell you how I shaved my legs to meet you?"

"Shaved your legs?" She rolls her eyes. "No, I can assure you that you never mentioned shaving your legs."

"Well, don't you want to know what shaving my legs has to do with meeting you?"

"I have a feeling that the story is forthcoming."

The first thing I did after hearing that Margaret B. Parkinson, executive editor of Bobbs-Merrill, would meet with me for fifteen minutes was shave my legs so that I could wear stockings for the first time in eight years. In Santa Cruz, where I lived, women did not shave their legs or underarms. If men didn't, women shouldn't. But after my mother remarked that I could begin braiding the hair on my legs any day now, I decided I would make a better impression if I shaved them. I bought a navy blue skirt at Loehmann's and borrowed a briefcase with the combination 0-0-0 from a friend. Into the briefcase I put Chapstick, a brush, and fifteen dollars.

Two months before our meeting, I had sent a four-page query letter to thirty editors at New York publishing houses. I included everything the 1980 *Writer's Market* suggested: why I thought an anthology about compulsive eating was original; why I considered myself capable of writing it; why the reading public needed this book now; why the editor should consider reading my manuscript as soon as possible. Twenty-nine rejection letters arrived over the next three weeks. Sorry, we're not interested, sorry, this book is not for us, sorry. I remembered what my writing teacher told us about rejections: wallpaper your bathroom with them, don't take them personally, keep sending out your work. I remembered what my father said when he heard I wanted to write a book: What makes you think you're different from thousands of starving writers who try for years to get their work published? Do you know, my father said, that someone sent Charles Dickens's work (under a different name, of course) to a publisher and was turned down? Forget writing, he said. Go to law school, he said.

On a Tuesday in March, I received a letter from an editor at Bobbs-Merrill: "Dear Ms. Roth: I found your idea quite interesting. Please send me your manuscript. Yours, Margaret B. Parkinson, Executive Editor."

After the ecstasy died down, I remembered something pivotal: In the query letter I had stated I had a manuscript, and I didn't. I had an idea for a manuscript—an anthology by women on hunger, nourishment, starving ourselves, bingeing, breaking free from compulsive eating. I had been collecting short stories, poems, and journal pieces for three years. But all I had was three hundred file folders with writers' names, the titles of their pieces, and possible chapter titles. Lying and not having a manuscript were admittedly not the best way to begin a relationship with a publisher, but with the support of my writing group, I called Peg's office before my annual Passover trip to New York and arranged with her secretary, Mercedes, to have a fifteen-minute meeting with her.

It was a crazy dream, to be a writer. I'd heard the Charles Dickens line from my friend Elizabeth, my aunt Rose, and the woman who sold Peruvian lilies at the stand across the street from Gayle's Bakery. Each time the story was told, a different writer had gotten his work rejected. So far Ernest Hemingway, Leo Tolstoy, and William Faulkner wouldn't have gotten published if they lived today, so why not save myself the anguish? Even my best friend, Sara, looked at me askance when I said I was writing a book. "You and how many other people?" she said. But I didn't want to do anything else. I had already been an astrologer, a chemist, a maid, a dishwasher, a counselor in a Suicide Prevention and Crisis Service. I had been a saleswoman in an art gallery, an encounter-group leader, a switchboard operator, a waitress, a nursery school teacher, an avocado and cheese sandwich maker for a local health food store. I had worked at those jobs because I had to, because I needed the money. But I was always tapping my foot, watching the clock, feeling defeated, because I knew there was something I could be doing that would tie purple ribbons around my heart. I was fired from one job because of insolence, left the others because of boredom. When, at twenty-eight, I took six months off between jobs, I told myself I could do whatever I wanted to do, however impractical it seemed. An old gray horse called Writing came loping out of childhood dreams.

In Mrs. Epstein's fifth-grade class, our first writing assignment had been to tell a story about something magical. I sat on my bed that night with two pieces of white lined paper resting on top of the *World Book Encyclopedia* and began writing. A story flew out. I wrote on the bumpy red book as fast as I could, describing the images that paraded in back of my eyes, one following another. A girl named Tammy flies on a plane to San Antonio, Texas, and all the stewardesses get sick and no one knows what to do. The cabins are in chaos until Tammy and her dog, Dot, take over. They serve meals, talk to the elderly people, play with the children. They become national heroes, get medals of honor.

When I read the story to the class the next day, I stepped out of the things that usually mattered to me— my fighting parents, my anxiety at what was going to happen between them, my fat thighs. For a few minutes it didn't matter what Robert Maguire or Ricky Ashford thought of me. I had created something that didn't exist the day before, from a place that didn't belong to anyone but me. I started keeping a journal, started writing poetry, short stories. I never showed anyone what I wrote. I was so frightened that someone would tell me I shouldn't or couldn't do it that I wrote secretly, in journals with locks and keys, and in poems that I hid in my socks drawer. By the time I was twenty-eight, I had twenty journals, a manuscript I had written when John Kennedy was shot, and poems about parakeets, broken hearts, and divorce. The thought of being published, of traversing the distance from my socks drawer to a bookstore, was inconceivable. Then I joined a writing group, and they encouraged me to see the executive editor at Bobbs-Merrill.

Margaret B. Parkinson was standing behind her desk with her hand extended. Hello, Geneen, I'm Peg Parkinson. Sit down. I noticed how skinny she was. I noticed the three-foot soft-sculpture pencil hanging above her desk. Then I sat down and told myself to breathe.

I forced myself to look at her, really look. She was wearing a navy blue V-neck sweater with a chunky brass necklace around her neck. On her hand was an antique diamond ring, two emerald-cut diamonds in a platinum S setting. Her hair was cropped short and hung in soft waves of gray and brown around her long, weathered face. Deep lines around her eyes and forehead, at the corners of her mouth and above it, spoke of hard living. But her eyes looked amused behind what was supposed to be a very professional demeanor.

"Tell me about your book," she said as she picked up a cigarette that was burning in an ashtray. The curls of smoke formed a soft blue curve between us. I suddenly knew that she was kind—I could tell by the way she looked at me, the way she sat, the way she held her cigarette, the amusement in her eyes—and that she was genuinely interested in who I was, what I was doing. I didn't plan what I said next. I opened my mouth and let the blue haze between us absorb the words. I told her about the women in my workshops, my own struggle with food, the fact that no one had written about being a compulsive eater from the compulsive eater's point of view.

She crushed her cigarette in the green glass ashtray, leaned forward in her chair. "I love your idea," she said, "but anthologies don't sell well. The reader needs to identify with one voice throughout the book—so you will need to write at least half of it. You'll need to write introductions to all the chapters, and you'll need to write pieces of your own to put in the chapters. This needs to be your book; the reader needs to feel that she knows you, your struggle, your triumphs with food."

I nodded, mute. I didn't want to tell her that I had only planned to include one of my poems in the book and to write the introduction. Just as my writing teacher, Ellen Bass, had done in her anthology, *No More Masks*. This book was my way of getting my feet wet in the publishing world, not a chance to dive in headfirst. Her suggestion thrilled me a fraction more than it terrified me.

Peg continued: "Do you know how long it takes to produce a book once it is accepted?" I shook my head no. "About as long as a pregnancy—nine months. Once you hand in the manuscript, I will edit it, go over it with you, and then it goes to copy, layout, typesetting, et cetera. So, when can I see it?"

My heart was racing, and my mother's white silk blouse was sticking to my back. I told her that I would go home and begin writing the chapter introductions, that I would send her a chunk of the book in two weeks.

"Don't put this off, Geneen," she said, standing up. "This is a fabulous idea, and if you don't do it, someone else will."

"I won't," I said. By now I felt as if I had walked into

someone else's life, someone who was used to meetings like this in places like this with people like this. Someone who knew what to say next. Something witty, something brilliant, something literary.

"That's a great pencil," I finally said, pointing to the soft-sculpture pencil above her desk.

"Thanks," she said. "A friend gave it to me. It's one of my most prized possessions. It reminds me that publishers need writers. Sometimes we get carried away with ourselves, feel very important, treat writers as if you are not important—but you are. Remember that—and send me that book soon."

Back in California, I sat at my kitchen table and tried to write.

Nothing.

I told myself that I could write through the nothing, keep my pen moving, and that it was okay to write "I don't know what to write" a hundred times. But after a few hours I'd go to the refrigerator, eat some frozen cake, look outside the window at the calle lilies, and decide that tomorrow would be better. It wasn't. Every day I'd get up with a resolve to begin the first chapter introduction, and every day I'd spend three or four hours with nothing to say.

Peg called two weeks after my meeting with her.

"Well, Geneen? How's it going?"

"Fine. I'm moving right along on these introductions."

"Good, good. This is going to be an important book. Call me if you have any questions or need any help."

"Thanks, Peg, I will."

I couldn't believe she had called me. I couldn't believe she cared about my book. I couldn't believe I couldn't write. I had been writing every day during the past three years. I had a stack of poems, two short stories, a piece that was being published in an anthology, a poem that was being published in a newspaper. I never had any problems with blocks. And now that a New York City editor was actually interested, I couldn't write a word.

Peg kept calling. Every two weeks she'd ask me how it was going, and every two weeks I'd answer fine. I didn't want her to lose hope, to stop believing in me or the book.

After two months of not writing and lying to her, I wrote the following letter:

Dear Peg,

Thank you so much for your interest in my book. I can't tell you how much it means to me that you believe in this project. I didn't think that editors got as involved with their writers as you have gotten with me, and it's cheered me tremendously to feel you so present.

But I have something I must tell you: I've been lying to you since my return from New York. I haven't written a word on the book, and for some reason I can't write. I guess there is something about being published that is too frightening to me. In any case, I am ashamed of myself for lying to you. When I wrote that query letter, I never thought anyone would be interested in it, and now that you are, I can't seem to proceed with confidence or even dignity. I thought I wanted to be a writer, but I was wrong. So, please accept my sincere apology. I am withdrawing my idea for the book, and will get on with my life as a non-writer. You've been wonderful. Any writer would be fortunate to have you as an editor.

I walked to the Seabright Avenue post office and opened the blue box, put the letter in, closed the box, cried. I didn't have it in me to be a writer. I didn't have poetic words and creative ways to put them together. I couldn't even remember what the word *desultory* meant. I didn't have stories running around in my head that I just had to express. And I couldn't function under pressure. Maybe the truth was that I wanted to be a writer because I couldn't hold down any other kind of job. I didn't know. I only knew that I didn't want to sit at my kitchen table anymore eating frozen cake and pretending that something original was lurking inside my brain, my heart, and if I tried long enough, would spill onto the paper in front of me.

Five days after I mailed the letter, I received a phone call from Peg. When I first heard her voice, I thought she was calling to yell at me for lying to her.

"Hello, Geneen, this is Peg."

"Peg? Oh, God, I didn't expect to hear from you. You must be furious with me."

"Geneen, I'm not giving up on you."

"What?"

"I know you must be very frightened to write a letter like that, but I believe in you and I believe in your book.

I know you can do this. I know you can write a terrific book and that the world will eat it up."

"Peg—"

"No Pegs about this. I know this is true. And I know that when you are ready to do it, you will. Here's my number at home. You already have my number at the office. Call me collect anytime, day or night, if I can help you. And send me the book when it's done. You can do this. Just take it easy and do it at your own pace."

I heard a click and then a dial tone. Phone in hand, I sat there, stunned. She wasn't angry. She thought I could do this. She believed in me. I put the phone in the cradle, sat staring out the window. I realized immediately that her call had freed me. I had needed to know that her interest would not rob me of the only thing in the world that was mine, my words, my thoughts. I needed to know that if I wrote the book, it would be for me, not for her. I sat down the next day and started to write. Six weeks later, I walked to the Seabright Avenue post office, opened the blue box, and mailed the complete manuscript. Then I went home and called Peg.

"Well, dearie, how are you?"

"Fine. I'm calling to tell you some exciting news."

"And what might that be?"

"I just mailed the manuscript. You should be receiving it in a few days."

"Now, where have I heard this before?"

"No, honestly, Peg, I'm telling the truth."

"I'll believe it when I see it."

We talked about summer in New York, how hot, how

miserable it was; she told me about her garden in East Quogue, about the Sea Foam roses she had planted and the Burmese Honeysuckle that was budding on her deck. She didn't believe I had sent the manuscript, and because I knew I had, I could afford to laugh about the situation. I teased her about not believing me; she teased me about crying wolf.

Five days later, she called again.

"I love it."

"Peg?"

"I stayed up all night reading it, and all I can say is every time a piece of yours came to the end, I wanted more. I want more Geneen Roth. She is a fine writer."

"You really think so?"

"I'm not prone to exaggeration. You wrote a good book, Geneen."

"Thank you. And thanks for believing in me, Peg."

She took a drag on a cigarette. "Oh, now don't get all mushy on me. You're the one who wrote it."

"Yeah, and you're the one who stood on the sidelines and cheered."

"Enough about that—when can you come to New York?"

A month later, I walked into the Bobbs-Merrill office on Fifty-seventh Street and Fifth Avenue. The book was then called "Is There Life After Chocolate?" When I walked into the reception area, the receptionist was wearing a button with a blue elephant saying "Things

Are Getting Worse. Please Send Chocolate." When she called Peg on the phone to say I was waiting, Mercedes came out wearing a chocolate button. She brought me into Peg's office, where I saw a button on the stuffed pencil and a bowl of chocolate kisses. Peg was sitting behind her desk, reading a manuscript. She was wearing a pearl gray cardigan sweater with a white blouse, and large earrings, goldish triangles, that emphasized her long, thin face. A cigarette was smoking in the green ashtray. When she saw me, she smiled a quick, lopsided smile, dismissed the buttons with a wave of her hand, as if to say that anyone would make her staff wear buttons with elephants and chocolate. She stood, extended her hand. "How's the girl writer today?" she asked.

"Excited," I answered.

"How about hungry?"

We walked down Fifty-seventh Street to Gaylord's Indian restaurant. It was dark and smelled of saffron. People were dressed in gray suits with red polka-dot ties and speaking in hushed tones. Sitar music was playing, and I felt as if I were in a movie. I ordered vegetable curry with onion naan; Peg ordered tandoori chicken and a half bottle of champagne. When we toasted, she said, "We want to buy your book and publish it next fall." I squealed and then tried to sound sophisticated, respectable. "That's wonderful, Peg. I'm so pleased you like my book."

She told me about editing, copy editing, designing a cover, the sales conference, the sales force selling it to the stores. A fortune-teller dressed in a blue pleated caftan with a gold turban on his head walked to our table and asked if we would like our fortunes told. Peg nodded yes and then said to me, "Why don't you let this gentleman tell you how rich and famous you are about to become?" He pulled up a chair and sat down next to me, took my palm in his hand, and said, "You are about to embark on a wondrous journey" to which Peg replied, "Yah, and we're about to pay for it."

I laughed a loud, nervous laugh that made the polka-dot ties turn in my direction as the fortune-teller walked to the next table. I wanted to say something brilliant, but I couldn't think of anything beyond the usual questions of what other books she had edited, where she had worked before. I wanted Peg to be glad she had accepted my book, to think I was smart. She wasn't like anyone I had ever known. She used words like desultory and rutilant. She quoted Shakespeare and E. M. Forster (if food be the music of love, play on . . .), went to chamber music concerts at the Ninety-second Street Y and was the kind of New Yorker that had never been, or had any desire to go, to California. To Peg, California was filled with people who ate granola, wore Birkenstocks, and named their children Rainbow and Mountain (promise me, she said years later, that you won't name your child Rock or Sunset. No natural phenomena).

Back in the Bobbs-Merrill office, Peg said she would be in touch, that she'd have an edited version of the manuscript in about three weeks and we would go over it together. She told me that this book was the first in a long line of books for me. She called me Lambchop. She said, "I'm about to do something, heaven forbid, they do in California." She hugged me good-bye.

Two weeks after I returned home, I received a phone call. "Geneen? This is Peg..." Her voice sounded slurred, as if the words had fallen together and she couldn't unglue them.

"Hi, Peg," I said tentatively.

"I have something to tell you, Geneen, something I'm very, very sorry about." She sounded as if she was going to cry, and I thought, this is it, she decided she doesn't like my book, the whole thing has been a giant mistake and she's taking it all back, I knew it, I knew it. "I'm an alcoholic, Geneen, and I was drunk the day we went out to lunch. I shouldn't have done that, I should have told you. I'm really sorry."

I was silent. I didn't know what to say. "Don't worry about it, Peg, it's fine" or "Does this mean you don't like my book?" or "What effect does this have on you, our relationship, your job?" or "You didn't look drunk, are you sure?" I didn't understand why she was telling me and what she needed from me. But I suddenly understood why she was so interested in my work: it was about a subject she knew well—the siren call of addiction.

"Are you drunk now, Peg?"

"Yes."

That was the first of a long series of drunk conversations I had with her, when I didn't know that it was no use to talk to her then, that she wouldn't remember anything either of us said, that she said things she didn't mean. We got off the phone, and I was ashamed of myself. For allowing myself to have big dreams. For thinking that anyone sober could believe I had something to say.

Two days later she called again. "I am an alcoholic," she said, "but I am working on it, and I shouldn't have called you. Sometimes the pain gets too much. I am well aware of the liabilities of drinking, so please, no lectures."

"Okay. No lectures."

"Did I say anything terribly awful?" she asked.

"No, not terrible. You used the word fuck a few times. You told me about a homeless woman that lives at the end of your block. You talked about South Africa, and you said fuck a few more times. That's about it."

"Well, let's forget that abominable incident and move on to a much happier topic—your book."

We talked about some poems that she thought should not be included in the book. "I want this book to be for everyone," she said, "and although I love poetry, I want this book to be readable like a novel, the kind of book you can't put down, the kind you want to stay up all night and read. But if you feel strongly about keeping them in, I will defer to you. It is your book, and you should have the last word always."

I didn't feel strongly. In the ten years I worked with Peg, I disagreed with her editorial opinion only once— when she told me that hate was too strong a word to use for the way compulsive eaters felt about themselves. I told her that hate was mild, that there wasn't a word strong enough to describe the feeling.

When *Feeding the Hungry Heart* had been in the stores for three months, Peg called me and told me it was time to write my second book. I told her I wasn't ready. I needed time off; I needed to discover my own rhythm again. She told me I needed to get off my ass. She said, "One book is a fluke. But when you write two books, people know you are serious." I said I didn't care whether people knew I was serious. I knew I was serious. She said she would call me in a week.

Exactly seven days later, she called and asked if I had changed my mind. Was I ready to write the next book? I said of course not. And anyway, what did she think I should write this book on? She said, compulsive eating. She said, you let people know that there is a way out. *Feeding the Hungry Heart* was descriptive. Now you need to write a prescriptive book. You need to let people know what the way out is, she said. What about my poetry? I said. What about it? she said. You'll get back to it after you've published two books. No, I said, and that's final. I don't want to repeat myself, I said. I'll call you in a week, she said.

Seven days and two hours later, Peg called. Geneen, she said, enough messing around. I know you don't want to be caught in the niche of compulsive eating for the rest of your life, but what you did is not fair, it really isn't. You have a social responsibility to the women whose lives you touched. Would it really take so much for you to write another book? You could do it in a year, and then your job would be done. Besides, do you have anything specific in mind that you want to be writing? Why not write this in the meantime? Writers write, Geneen. And this is as good as anything else to spend your time on.

I'll think about it, I said.

Good, I'll call you in a week.

My friend Jill came for tea the next day. I told her about Peg's calls and that I wasn't ready to begin another book so soon. I didn't want to be commissioned for a book. I wanted to think of the idea and let it evolve over time, the way *Feeding the Hungry Heart* had.

She raised her eyebrows. She said, Michelangelo was commissioned to paint the Sistine Chapel. And then she took a sip of jasmine tea.

I thought about it constantly for the next few days. I knew that what Peg was saying about writing a prescriptive book was true, that I hadn't been specific about how to climb out of the obsession with food. And I felt passionate about the subject. I had more to say, much more. But I wanted to be a real writer; I wanted my life to match the images in my head. Images of being agonized, smoking cigarettes, drinking scotch. Wandering around in a haze of cigarette smoke and abandon while I cranked out words on a small black manual typewriter. Male writers haunted my dreams: Fitzgerald, Carver, Hemingway. The self-destruction, the drama, the great art, while the women in their lives went unnoticed, unmet, or crazy.

In the end, I chose to believe Peg because she believed in me. If I doubted part of what she said, the kind of book I should write, then I would have to doubt it all—that my voice counted. So I started cranking out words on my gray Olympia typewriter, and she continued to wander in a haze of cigarette smoke and alcohol.

When I gave her the first four chapters on my next visit to New York, she called my hotel room three hours later and left a message saying, "The manuscript is good enough to eat."

Months would go by when we talked every week or so, checking in. She'd tell me about her house in 'East Quogue, her garden, her cat Queen Elizabeth. Then I wouldn't hear from her for a few weeks, and I would call her. The phone would ring three, four, five times. She'd pick it up. "Helllllooooo?" and I'd hear the slurred voice, the whimpering. I'd beg her to stop drinking, ask her to come live with me for a month and dry out. I'd send her flowers, information about AA, pamphlets about Smoke Enders. On a sober day, after our hellos and talk about her doctor telling her she must stop smoking because of her emphysema, I said, "You're killing yourself, Peg."

"Oh, stop being so melodramatic. I know I should stop smoking, and I have cut down. And I can't stand those AA meetings. Everyone slobbering over everyone else. I'm going to take Anabuse. I'm taking care of it, don't worry, Geneen. Get cracking on that book. That's the only thing you need to worry about. I'm a big girl. I can take care of myself."

"Yes, but why would someone who has emphysema smoke cigarettes if she didn't want to kill herself?"

"Because she likes the taste of cigarettes. Like someone I know who likes the taste of chocolate—"

"Chocolate is not killing me."

"That's why I want you to write this book. So that you can tell people who *are* killing themselves with chocolate how to stop killing themselves."

When I called to tell her the finished manuscript was on its way, she was drunk. She told me to fuck off, and then she told me about the homeless woman who lived down the block from her apartment. "She doesn't have a place to sleep. She doesn't have any money," Peg said, crying. "I must give her some. She doesn't have any food. I must give her some, I must give her some—"

"Do you have any alcohol in the house now, Peg? Are you still drinking?" I asked.

"Under my bed. But you don't understand, she doesn't have any. I must give her some money."

"Peg, I'll call you tomorrow." I hung up. I called her friend Annie. I told her that Peg needed help, and could she please go to her apartment? I was furious with Peg and ashamed of myself for being furious. I couldn't believe this was the person responsible for my book. I wanted to fly to New York, kick her in the ass, shake her by the shoulders and tell her to get her act together.

Then I began a rapid descent into the land of what's

wrong with me. The litany went like this: My writing is the kind of writing only a drunk could like; I should have known she was drunk that first day at Gaylord's, and I should have done something then (what, though? I couldn't figure that part out). I feel as if I am back in my family, completely dependent on a crazy person. Of all the editors in the world, I wind up with one that makes me feel like a child again. I knew this was too good to be true.

Three weeks later, I received the edited book in the mail with a note of apology from Peg. "Forgive me, please. Your book is very good indeed." As I flipped through the manuscript, I began to laugh, despite my anger with her. In a paragraph about feeling beautiful, she responded: "G—your mother and Sara and I know you're beautiful, but the reader will feel it's unbecoming of you to keep pointing it out." Next to a paragraph about playing with food, she wrote, "I think this is just too dumb for words, but it's your book, and if you want it, it stays. But please fix in some sensible way." A large X was drawn through what I thought was my most poetic metaphor of the book, hands waving, reaching, asking for food. Beside it she wrote, "I think it's time to wave bye-bye to these tiny hands."

On green slips of paper pasted to the page, her comments made me respect the elegance of language, think deeply about what I was saying, giggle at my ignorance or arrogance. She made me feel as if she remembered the heart of what I wanted to say when I had forgotten it, and that it was her work to hold that vision. She was not going to let me take shortcuts. She was not going to let me trivialize or cheapen the language. She was going to keep pushing until I remembered, grew into my original dream for the piece, came back to where I started. I never felt as if she was trying to change my voice, only to take away the frills and the artifice so that its sound would be true. I handed her some pieces I hadn't dared show anyone, some I was embarrassed by, some I was proud of, some I was uncertain of. She never laughed at me. With a practiced ear she heard when I was trying to sound like Virginia Woolf or Ernest Hemingway. She'd write, "Virginia, this worked better in *To the Lighthouse*." She handed me a truer version of my work than the one I handed her. And because her skill prevented her from injecting her voice, her thoughts, I kept becoming larger in her presence, kept returning to who I would have been without the pretense of who I thought I should be.

I realized then what a privilege it was to know her, to have her in my life, drunk or sober. And I wanted to return the gift. When someone who didn't steal it gives your wandering heart back to you, anything you can do in return seems like small potatoes.

I tried harder to get through. I decided that I wouldn't hold back my feelings about her because she squirmed under an affectionate gaze. When she lost her job at Bobbs-Merrill, I tried to find her other jobs. During the next few years I kept writing, I kept sending her my pieces to edit. When I wrote a book proposal, she sent it back to me and stated, "Try again. This doesn't work. You're not saying anything new. I'm afraid you'll think I've dealt too harshly with you. Talk to you next week—xoxoP." A few months later, I sent her a new proposal, and she called, left a message on the machine. "This is absolutely wonderful. You've finally hit on something that feels right. Go to it, girl." Then, as the book was based on meeting Matt and my relationship to him, she wrote Matt a letter:

Dear Matthew:

Well, thank *goodness*! First of all for making Geneen settled and happy and looking forward to your dual future.

But also for giving her the book she's been wanting to write. I felt bad about not being able to encourage her on other ideas, but this one feels right and is.

I'm just as pleased as can be—

Love,
Peg

Every time I called her, I'd hold my breath until she answered. I never knew whether she would be sober and working at her desk, or drunk and passed out on her bed. Everything she was, she was in excess: funny, sensitive, tough, brilliant, kind, self-destructive. After the first year with her, I knew that one day her extremes would collide, and she'd go up like dry sticks in a blaze. I knew hers was a life that would not see old age. And I knew any thoughts I had about saving her life were grandiose. The only thing I could do was love her, and hope that I was wrong about the blaze.

I wasn't.

Nine years after I met Peg she was diagnosed with liver cancer. She spent a few months in and out of hospitals, receiving chemotherapy. I was writing *When Food Is Love*, and instead of waiting to send her the completed manuscript, I sent it to her chapter by chapter. Her revisions became short, and her writing became shaky. I cherished her comments nevertheless, put them in a large manila envelope close by so that I could hear her voice, refer to it again and again.

When she died in the hospital, her friend Victoria told me that a letter I had written to her was next to her bed. And that she had read it every few days during those last weeks.

A year before she was diagnosed with cancer, I had dedicated a book to her, and with the dedication I had written a letter:

Meeting you changed everything.
... If you ever feel that you haven't accomplished enough in your life, I want you to remember that you gave at least one person—me—what many people die without ever knowing: the grounded-in-my-body knowledge that who I am and what I have to say is worth something. I love you, Peg. You live inside me forever.

At her memorial service, I spoke of our first meeting, the letter I had written about the lies I had spoken. I described some of her funniest editorial comments. The time she filled in the blank of a workbook in which I gave an example of making a cake in the shape of the Empire State Building. Peg wrote, "If you leave this in, I will jump off the top." Other friends spoke of her kindness to strangers, how she fed plumbers, electricians, homeless women. I cried at the service, and then I didn't cry again. She'd say that my tears were sentimental slop and that she'd had her life, she'd done what she did with it, to get on with my own. To keep writing. One of the last things she said to me was, "Hasn't your Auntie Peg taught you anything? When will you ever learn the difference between lie and lay?"

Probably never.

After the memorial service I asked her friend Selma if I could have one possession of Peg's, the treasure that had followed her from Bobbs-Merrill to Madison Avenue to East Quogue.

It hangs above my desk now, a three-foot pencil on a green string.

Chapter Five

■

WOMEN'S FRIENDSHIPS: A CONSPIRACY OF HUNGER

■

The first time I met Sara, I was wearing pink satin shoes with soles as thin as pancakes. My boyfriend, Tom, had given them to me for my twenty-eighth birthday the week before, and wearing them made me feel brave, willing to risk the grease marks of life.

When I knocked on the door, a woman appeared dressed in a black-and-white-striped shirt, black pants, black-and-white-striped socks, and black-and-white-checked earrings. Her hair was wavy and, like her clothes, was black and white. "I'm Sara," she said, extending her hand, "come in." We walked through a living room with a baby grand piano and entered a small room lined with books and two butterscotch leather chairs facing each other. Sara stood behind one of the chairs and pointed at the other, said, "Please sit down."

I sat in the chair opposite her, waiting.

She eased into the chair, straightened her black and white shirt, crossed her legs, gave me a wise, reassuring look. Took a deep breath.

"Tell me why you've come."

Another look. Another breath. Then: "How can I help you?"

I remembered hearing that she was a therapist, and realized that she assumed I'd come for a counseling session. In fact, I had come to meet with her husband, Cliff, about making a desk. I considered going through with the session, telling her about my troubles with Tom, so that I wouldn't have to embarrass her. Then I realized that although I'd done some ridiculous things in my life to avoid causing someone discomfort, this would be going too far. I tried to model the wisdom and compassion I saw on her face before I spoke, tried to let her know that although she had just made a complete fool of herself, her life didn't have to end here.

"I'm afraid there's been a slight mix-up," I said haltingly. "I have a meeting with your husband to design a desk."

Her face went blank, then registered disbelief. Two rows of small teeth peeked out of her mouth in a broad smile. "Well," she said, "I guess this is one of life's most embarrassing moments, because I am thoroughly and absolutely embarrassed."

She giggled, a high three-note trill that reminded me of the day school let out for summer, and in that moment I knew we would be friends.

We met for tea a few times at the café behind the bookstore. We talked for hours and parted reluctantly. After

our fourth meeting Sara suggested that we give ourselves
the luxury of regular weekly dates.

On Tuesday afternoons, dressed in some kind of
matching skirt-socks-earrings combination (usually black
and white, usually checks and stripes), Sara rang the bell,
and we sat at the table drinking tea, talking. At some
point the chairs got too hard, so we moved to the emerald green and burgundy futons on the living room floor.
After a few months of Tuesdays, we skipped the chairs
and started out on the floor, spending hours talking, telling the stories of our lives, as light webbed through the
cream lace curtains.

We fell in love the way women fall in love with their
friends. Like Russian dolls, one inside the other, the
mother becoming the child who becomes the mother of
the child. Endlessly falling into each other, then separating, falling, then separating. We were like starfish growing new parts, extending new selves, as if in meeting
each other, we had the chance to reinvent ourselves, to
rearrange ourselves, to become whole.

With Sara, I had a feeling of profound welcome; our
friendship seemed to turn the seasons, fill the hollow,
burnt places in me. It was the reflection of womanness
that was so satisfying. The way I seemed to know her im-
pulses, her reasons, what she was reaching for. The way
she knew me, could hold the vision of who I wanted to
be despite who I believed myself to be at that moment.

Our fundamental sameness contrasted with the thousands of ways we were different. She was grounded in
home; I traveled constantly. She worked at keeping her

life steady; I worked at keeping mine dramatic. She was social, extroverted, became enlivened around groups of people; I was reclusive, introverted, withered without time alone. Apart, we were small, separate; together, we were the best of each of us, a whole, shimmering world.

We started talking to each other every day, then a few times a day, started stopping in at each other's houses. Within six months neither of us could remember not knowing each other, what our lives were like before we met. We felt lucky, blessed, forever changed.

For ten years I looked at Sara and saw nothing but patience and compassion, wisdom and kindness, generosity and love. Most especially, I saw selflessness, a quality I was certain I lacked.

From year eleven to year thirteen, I looked at Sara and saw the most manipulative, vindictive, controlling person I'd ever known.

Beginning with year fourteen, two years ago, I looked at Sara and, for the first time, saw Sara.

The change of feelings after ten years of best friendship was precipitated (but not caused) by my move from Santa Cruz to Berkeley, seventy-five miles away, a move that Sara and I had talked about for two years prior to its happening. If you had asked, we would have told you that we knew that living in different cities would change our relationship, and were consciously mourning the passing of an era. We would have told you that we were sophisticated about feelings and owning our individual parts in conflicts; we prided ourselves on being able to work through sticky, messy situations. Moving an hour and a half away seemed difficult, but do-able—best friends survived worse (moves across the country, across the world) all the time.

Six weeks after I left Santa Cruz, my relationship with Sara fell apart. She told me she was frightened of driving long distances and would not visit me in Berkeley. She liked things the way they were, and since I was the one who had messed them up, I should be the one who made them better: She felt it was my job to come to Santa Cruz, not hers to come to Berkeley. She accused me of replacing her with my house, said I put too much energy into creating beautiful spaces, and that my house had become my new best friend. (We giggle about that now, but at the time it wasn't funny.) She said outrageous things, demanded outrageous gifts, became someone I didn't know, didn't like, was a breath away from hating.

I was stunned by her behavior, and I did what I used to do as a child when my mother backed me up against the wall with both her arms swinging: I became very still, dove to a place inside where she could not touch me, reach me, or hurt me. I felt victimized and betrayed, and wondered what I ever saw in this madwoman I once called my best friend.

We tried therapy. It didn't work. I tried doing forgiveness meditations. They helped, but only for a few hours. I tried reasoning with her about her "eye for an eye" theory. It was useless. She tried to convince me that she was right and I was wrong. I didn't believe her. Our hearts were raw and bleeding, and neither of us wanted more. Two and a half years after I moved to Berkeley, I wrote Sara a letter saying that I wanted to end our friendship.

I am leading a workshop in San Francisco, and we are making lists. I write the words, "Thin women are . . ," at the top of the flip chart, and ask the participants (ninety percent of whom are women) to call out endings to the sentence, to say whatever comes into their minds without censoring.

Thin women are . . .
stuck up
prissy
bored
shallow
superficial
only concerned with their looks
mean
insensitive
controlling
hungry
surrounded by men
self-confident

We make another list.

Fat women are . . .
lonely

sad
out of control
pathetic
willing to do anything to get thin
good listeners
sensitive
practiced at looking below the surface
deep
good at eating their feelings

And another.
If I were thin, women would . . .
think I didn't want to be friends with them
be jealous
want to know my secret
talk about me behind my back
think I had it all together
betray me
be frightened that I wanted their men
protect themselves from me
think I was not like them
reject me

This, in a room filled with women who want to be thin.

A woman named Chloe says, "My friends and I spent years talking about nothing but food and diets. Then I started losing weight, and then I started losing friends. The very same friends I'd gone on diet after diet with. These friends didn't want to hear that I was eating what

I wanted and losing weight. They didn't want to deal with my thinner body. I feel so hurt. They were my *friends*. I thought they would be happy for me."

Another woman says, "When I lost weight, my friends tried to sabotage the weight loss. They would give food to me, and if I didn't want it, they'd persist. They'd tell me how delicious the piece of cake was, oohing and ahhing about the icing as I sat at my desk. They couldn't stand to see me thin when they were fat."

As she is talking, I notice a response to one of the graffiti exercises on the wall. To the heading, "In the cafeteria of life . . ." someone has written: "I will never have a big enough tray."

I will never get enough.

I will always be hungry.

I will always want.

I will never have.

It is not surprising that if we believe that we will never have a big enough tray, we will be envious, silently furious when a friend's tray looks as if it is spilling over. It is also not surprising that, in our desire to stay safe, we make unconscious, unspoken agreements with friends: I'll stay fat if you stay fat; I'll stay needy if you stay needy; I'll keep myself small so that you won't be threatened. When we break the agreements (by losing weight, changing jobs, telling the truth, moving), all hell breaks loose.

Although hell breaking loose is often precipitated by weight loss, the issue is not about being thin or fat. It's about the meaning we ascribe to them. It's about emptiness and hunger and true nourishment. It's about deprivation and scarcity and what we believe about abundance and permission to live a big life.

Being thin is a culturally agreed-upon symbol for power and happiness in a woman. If it wasn't thinness, it would be something else. When food was scarce, being fat was a symbol of wealth, beauty, and power. The question is not what we look like, but the hunger we are willing to tolerate as part of our daily lives, and the fact that many of us use our friends to perpetuate that hunger. When a friend challenges the conspiracy of hunger, we feel threatened and envious and betrayed. We feel victimized and abandoned and hateful. Rather than deal with the emptiness that her change has evoked, we focus the attention on her, want to turn back the clock. We'd rather she gain back the weight than become aware of how we keep ourselves hungry. We'd rather everyone go hungry than everyone be full. Not because we are terrible people and want to see loved ones suffer, but because we don't believe that what happened to them can happen to us. We've lost the connection to our true, spacious nature.

But only temporarily.

Matt told me a story he heard at a conference: A man and his neighbor both owned chickens. One day the neighbor was given a beautiful cow, which he grew to love and care for. The cow provided milk and butter and cheese, which he shared with his friend. But the man was envious that his neighbor had a cow and he didn't. One day he found a bottle, rubbed it, and the proverbial genie appeared.

The genie said, "I will grant you one wish, but only one. Think carefully, consider your life, and then ask me for anything you can imagine."

The man said, "Kill the cow."

And it was done.

He could have asked for a herd of cows. Or a farm with a garden *and* horses *and* sheep *and* cows. He could have asked for happiness or joy or sexual ecstasy forever, but all he wanted was to diminish the size of his neighbor's life rather than increase the size of his own.

When I moved to Berkeley and Sara reacted the way she did, I felt as if my best friend wanted to kill my cow.

I'd wanted to move for many years, but I didn't know where to go, and I didn't want to leave Sara. My life was getting smaller and smaller in Santa Cruz, although I couldn't exactly say why, and I didn't want to hurt Sara's feelings, so I never told her. When I met Matt, he moved to Santa Cruz for three years, until his Berkeley-based business needed his presence full-time. I agreed to move, for me, for him, and for us.

I lied to Sara and then felt betrayed because she wasn't supporting my growth or my happiness. I acted as if Matt and I needed to move for his business, which was true, and that I didn't have a choice, which was not true. I did the same thing with Sara that I had done with my mother: I shape-shifted. I knew what would please her and what would anger her, and I kept the parts of myself that would anger her out of our relationship.

There were good reasons for doing this with my mother. One of them is that it insured my survival. There are no good reasons for doing this with friends. Except that, six years ago, I still believed that lying was a compassionate response to Sara's pain, and that my life depended on hiding myself.

One of the Breaking Free eating guidelines is to "eat with the intention of being in full view of other people." This doesn't mean, as I tell people in a workshop, that if you live alone, you drag people off the street to watch you eat. It means that if someone walks in the door while you are eating, you don't swallow quickly, and stash the plate of mashed potatoes under the covers or pretend it was for the dog. It means that you allow people to see what you eat, even if you weigh three hundred pounds and are bingeing on cream puffs and chocolate cherries, because when you hide, you give yourself the message that who you are is not acceptable, and that you must pretend to be someone else to be loved, someone who eats chicken without skin and salad without dressing instead of cream puffs and chocolate-covered cherries. When you sneak food, you perpetuate the belief that you are too ugly, too needy, too intense to be seen and loved for who you are.

The same is true when you sneak feelings. The way I did with Sara. But the fact that I left Santa Cruz spoke for itself, the way losing weight speaks for itself. You can't hide the fact that you are thinner. (You could, I suppose, wear clothes that are three sizes too big, but that's not what most people want to do when they lose weight.) I couldn't hide the fact that I was leaving, and though I tried to shirk responsibility for it, leaving broke the conspiracy of hunger between Sara and myself, a conspiracy of which neither of us was consciously aware.

Another story, this one an old Sufi tale about Nasrudin the fool:

Nasrudin loses his keys in the house. A neighbor finds him crawling around on his hands and knees outside at night under a streetlamp.

"What are you doing, Nasrudin?" the neighbor asks.

"I am looking for my keys," he answers.

"Did you lose them here?"

"No, I lost them in the house."

"Why are you looking on the street when you lost them in the house?"

"Because," Nasrudin replies, "the light is better here than in my house."

Soon after we met, Sara and I agreed that we would look for our keys together. If one of us found the keys we'd lost, we'd keep looking until the other found hers. We also agreed that although we lost them inside the house, we would find them in the pockets of the other person. She was the key for me, and I for her; we were each other's answer. While it was acceptable to have other friends and a husband, it was the bond between us as women that counted most. We understood the trials of living with a man, of being a woman in a sexist society. We understood what it was like to bleed every month, to be afraid to walk alone at night, to want to talk about everything we saw, felt, believed. We understood each other the way no one else could; we needed each other to survive, and we would be true to this bond first and forever.

There are many problems with unconscious agreements like ours, but the main one is that it is based on deficiency and emptiness, hunger and scarcity. It is based on the belief that who I am is not enough, that in the cafeteria of life I will never have a big enough tray, and that my only chance for fulfillment lies outside myself. My only power resides in being able to figure out how to get enough from people and things around me.

Since the nature of deficiency is that nothing will ever be enough, no matter how much someone loves me, it doesn't stick. To have a continual experience of being worthy, I must have a continual inflow of love. If I want to be full, and who I am is fundamentally empty, then I must compromise myself. I must lie, I must hide, and if I am fortunate enough to meet someone who fills the tray, I must not threaten her.

Although this description sounds more like being in prison than being a friend, it is what most of us call friendship or marriage.

We act as if we are walking through the world carrying baskets, collecting pleasures, and still foraging for more, as if experiences are blackberries and when we collect enough love and pleasure, we believe we'll find rest. We will put up our pleasures for the winter, and spread them on cinnamon rolls when our lives are thundery and cold.

But there is no time to rest, no storing for the hunger to come, because we are always hungry now. There is no such thing as enough because we believe that our very being is not enough.

In the cafeteria of life, when we move from the stance of deficiency, it is impossible to have a big enough tray.

To have enough, we have to believe that we *are* enough.

And when we believe we are enough, what we have will no longer matter.

After three years of struggling with how merged we'd become, and two years of working to untangle ourselves from the mess we'd created, Sara and I are again best friends. It is a very different friendship than before. I do not lay my brokenness at her feet and expect her to put me together. I do not ask her to fill the holes in me. I do not go to her as a child goes to her mother, and there are times when I miss the comfort of our old ways. I miss believing that someone knows better than me. I miss being told what to do. That sounds ridiculous, I know, especially since if Matt tries to tell me what to do, I give him a withering look and tell him to mind his own business. But I missed having a mother, and Sara became a

stand-in. I missed having someone I could rely on, someone whose values I trusted and respected. And this is the
hard part: No one can give me what I missed with my
mother.

Like so many of us, I blamed myself for the craziness
in my family. I grew up doubting my value and looking
for someone to give it back to me. And although it was
comforting to find in Sara someone whom I trusted and
valued and respected, it was not regenerative to get myself back the way she chose to give me to me. Because no
matter how loving and kind her version of me was, it was
still *her* version, which made me dependent on her presence and staying in her good graces. This dependence
led to lies and sneaking and the reinforcement of a false
self because it required that I stay small and hungry, and
I am neither small nor hungry.

A teacher once told me that I project my goodness onto
other people and claim what I think is bad in myself, for
myself. It is as if I wrap my best self in a glowing planet
and hand it to a best friend, say to her, "Be the embod-
iment of my goodness, and when I doubt my essence, remind me of the glow."

After I moved, Sara refused to remind me of the glow,
and I felt bereft and angry. Eventually, I had faced my
own emptiness, the feeling that I am not enough. It is
not a one-time event, this coming face to face with emptiness. It is the ground from which I moved, the lie
around which my life was built.

But beyond that lie is another world. It's not a parallel life. It's not a world I ever imagined. It's not a world where I am famous and loved, or even happy. In this world I get myself back. Not because I have done something fabulous or have finally learned to be generous and unselfish and thin forever. I get myself back because I go back to myself.

I missed the experience of trust and respect. I missed the experience of value and joy. I missed the experience of compassion and love. Missing them made me feel deficient, and feeling deficient made me feel dependent on other people for the things I missed. But as my drama with Sara unfolded, I saw that she didn't have them, either. All this time I thought she had my keys in her pocket. I thought she had a big enough tray. But it's just that she had a different tray, and I equated different with bigger. I thought she could give me what she had, and then I would have enough. I never really saw her; I saw her only in relation to what I was missing and what she could give me.

Had I been able to see Sara, I would have understood that she was as busy filling her tray as I was filling mine. Our friendship was based on trades: I'll give you my piece of apple pie if you give me your cheesecake. I'll give you my chicken sandwich if you give me your Caesar salad. In the end, our trays and our lives were exactly the same size as when we began. I still felt needy and empty. And so did she.

There is no such thing as having a happy childhood

now because childhood depended on having big people around who could give us what we needed, and we cannot get back what we lost from anyone else. Even if we could, why would we want to? Their trays are as meager as ours, no matter what they look like from our perspective.

No one else has what we lost because no one took what we lost to begin with. Yes, it's true that having a father who was drunk or a mother who was abusive blocked the experience of safety or peace or love, but it wasn't *their* safety or peace or love that was blocked, it was ours. A drunk father made it impossible to feel the fullness of who we were because who he was was big and terrifying, and we needed him to survive. As children with troubled parents, we could not know ourselves without reference to someone else. And it is this reference that we think we still need to feel whole. But it is this very reference that blocks us from feeling whole because it keeps us looking outside, under the street lamp for our keys.

To find the keys, we have to go in the house. To get ourselves back, we have to go back to ourselves. There is no other way. Being famous or being thin or being healthy or being rich or being in love or being best friends does not confer wholeness on the recipients. We have to go back through the layers. We get to the wholeness by working with what's keeping us feeling whole. We get to the experience of trust and respect by working with how we block ourselves from feeling them. We find the keys by looking for them where we lost them.

This is an unlayering process, not a cure. There are no easy answers, no how-to's. But anyone can do it, anytime, anywhere. Because all it takes is a true understanding of what you want.

When you deeply understand something, a release happens, and from that release, change occurs. When I understood that Sara's tray was as small as mine, I stopped looking longingly at her tray.

A few years ago, I understood that I could define love as something I felt with certain people, with Matt and with Sara, with friends and with family, or I could know it as a quality of my own being. I could choose between the experience of giving my heart away to someone who was looking to give her heart away, or else feel the exquisite and delicate sweetness of my own heart melting in my chest.

Now there is no going back.

Now I want both: the experience of myself as whole, and friends with whom to share my life and explore the journey.

The conspiracy of hunger into which Sara and I entered was an either/or arrangement: Either I had her, with all the riches and costs of that friendship, or I had myself. Since being with myself meant feeling empty or feeling wrong or feeling unworthy, it was not a difficult choice.

Being with myself still, at times, means feeling empty or wrong or unworthy. But now I understand that there is nothing Sara or anyone else can do to fill the emptiness or right the wrongness or make me feel lovable. It's not as if I didn't give it my best shot. I did, for ten years. But the conspiracy was built on a lie, and the lie was that if I stayed small, I would be safe. If I did everything the friendship required, I would not be racked with emptiness. The lie was that one person can be another person's safety, love, value, truth.

Every one of us longs for the truth. We long to feel whole. We long to know ourselves, and to break out of this gravity-bound orbit in which we circle day after day. When any relationship is built on a lie, it will come apart as soon as one person understands that being larger is possible.

We need to build our friendships on truth and wholeness and expansiveness. We need friends who can be with us in our loneliness, not people who will cheer us up so that we don't feel it. We need friends who get furious with us when we are not being real or true to ourselves, not who get angry when we don't do what they want us to do. We need friends who are not afraid of our pain or our joy. We need friends who are not invested in the way we look, what we do or what we feel, who are willing to see us without reference to themselves. We need friends who are willing to break out of gravity-bound orbits and spin with us into the unknown.

And we need to become those friends ourselves.

The questions are always these: does this friendship lead you toward a fuller life or does it confine you? Does it bring you closer to your heart or take you further away? Does it open you or does it close you? Does it allow you to trust yourself further or does it make you frightened of yourself? Does it enlarge your life or does it make your life smaller?

When a friend is a real friend, she doesn't want to kill your cow. And you don't want to kill hers. Because when you kill someone's cow, you take something precious from her and all you end up with is a dead cow.

A few months ago, Sara received a phone call in the middle of the night. A woman's voice asked if this was the Sara who was described in *When Food Is Love*. She said it was. Then the woman began crying and apologizing for calling at three a.m. She said she was calling from New Hampshire, that she had tracked down Sara through my books. She said she needed a friend like the Sara I described, someone who was patient and compassionate and wise.

Sara talked to her for about twenty minutes and then asked if she had a therapist. She said she did, and promised that she'd call her first thing in the morning. As they were saying good-bye, she said, "Everyone needs a Sara."

Images of that woman haunted me for the next few days. I thought about the desperation she must have felt to call someone she didn't know in the middle of the night. Thought about the loneliness of needing a friend, and imagining that someone she read about in a book could be that friend, that fantasy friend who could fill in the holes and be there no matter what. It's comforting to believe she's out there, or even that we already know her.

But it's also infantilizing because it keeps us searching for the keys in a place we will never find them.

Everyone already has a Sara—the capacity to understand their own exquisite hearts—and without that Sara, nothing and no one will ever be enough.

Chapter Six

∎

TO HAVE OR
HAVE NOT:
NOURISHMENT
AND SELF-DENIAL

∎

It is Yom Kippur, and Matt and I are fasting. I haven't fasted since I was anorexic, when I used to drink diluted fruit juice for six weeks at a time and break the fast with a dozen donuts and a gallon of ice cream. But today I want to fast. Millions of Jews around the world are fasting, and I want to fast with them. They are in temple, praying, and I want to pray with them. Matt and I are on an island in the Pacific Northwest where a wooden sign welcomes ten different faiths; Jews are not on the list, so we take our prayer books and go into the forest.

Yom Kippur is the holiest Jewish holiday of the year. It is the last of the Ten Days of Awe, a time when our deeds of the past year are reviewed, and our fate for the upcoming year is determined. The traditional metaphor for Yom Kippur is that, depending on our recommitment to a path of decency and love, God might take His ledger and transfer our names from the Book of Death to the Book of Life. The contemporary view is that it is a day to assess and judge our lives, to assess the quality of our existence and commitments. Yom Kippur is a time to reflect, to ask for forgiveness for the hurts we have caused in the year. It is a time to pause and say one long blessing before the long, bountiful meal of the year.

We set out for our walk in the early morning, wearing white, as the books suggest, "to resemble the angels." After hiking up Mount Willis, we are breathless and wobbly, and decide to rest under a red alder tree. I open the red-and-yellow-checked backpack, take out the prayer book, and read the beginning of the Al Chayt, a testimony to, and confession of, our imperfections:

> *Because the relief of pain is built into its perception,*
> *I search within and remember when:*
> *I did not use my power;*
> *I did not see;*
> *I resisted change;*
> *I wouldn't risk;*
> *I was afraid of excitement;*
> *By these namings, I ask for the help that I long for,*
> *the curative help, the insight.*

I lean back on the tree, close my eyes, and think, "Guilty on all counts," especially the ones about resisting change, not risking, being afraid of excitement. I think about the running conversation with Matt about having children. When we met, we both said we didn't want children. Now he's changed his mind, which forces me to examine why I am so ambivalent about having a baby.

We said we weren't going to do it, my friends and I. We said we were going to be free women, travel the world, take our work seriously, not allow ourselves to be encumbered by wailing, runny-nosed children. And then, one by one, they capitulated. Every friend, with one exception, who said she wasn't going to have a child has a child. One of them, my friend Adrienne, is pregnant now with twin boys. (Every time I think of her having two babies instead of one, and of them being *boys*, I shudder. Sara's friend Marlo has two boys, nine and twelve—they race around the house, knocking vases over, shooting guns, playing war. "Hellions," Sara and I call them.)

And yet I have been dreaming about babies, looking longingly at baby buntings, painting babies with blond curly hair. The curls are Matt's contribution, though it worries me that between my fine, straight hair and Matt's coarse, curly hair, our child could have a thatch of tired Brillo. Matt says that hair should be the least of my worries. Number one should be that I am forty-three and have never been pregnant (although I never wanted to be); and number two should be that I had a Dalkon shield for a year, a Copper-T for three years.

My gynecologist says I could have scarred fallopian tubes. She wants me to take a hysterosalpinogram, a test in which they inject radioactive dye into your tubes and monitor its path. I tell her to give my body a chance, that Matt and I haven't even tried to get pregnant—I've been too sick. And then I wonder if I've been sick because I don't really want to get pregnant, if I'm dreaming about babies because soon I won't be able to have one, and I always want what I can't have. I tell myself that it's just pressure, that I want a baby because all my friends have children or that I am afraid of getting old, of having my heart dry up like a rattled milkweed pod, and am under the illusion that having a child will keep me young. I tell myself that if I haven't wanted a baby until now, it's a sign that I don't want one at all. I tell myself that I am not the mothering type.

And then I ask myself what the mothering type is.

She's a woman with rosy cheeks (a cross between the Breck girl and a Renoir nude) who likes baking, sewing, camping, going to soccer games, schlepping. A woman with boundless energy, a den mother type, a homemaker. Someone who knows herself well enough to make her child feel secure, wanted, brave. Someone who is willing not only to give of her life but give *up* her life—for a child.

As my mother gave up her life. And didn't.

Matt picks up the prayer book. Reads the next piece:

> *We violate that which is Eternal when we violate ourselves; for our failures of truth, we ask for honesty and courage:*
>
> *For acting out of fear of looking at ourselves deeply and honestly;*
>
> *And for using honest self-examination as a substitute for changing ourselves.*

For paralyzing ourselves by thinking we could not change;

And for using these prayers as a substitute for real change.

For perpetuating vindictiveness by not forgiving our parents for the hurts they inflicted on us as children;

And for sustaining guilt and anxiety by not forgiving ourselves for the negative traits we inherited.

For giving ourselves to the fleeting pleasure of inflicting lasting hurts;

And for cynicism which eats away our faith in the possibility of love.

In naming these errors, I confront them, I accept them, and I commit myself to avoiding them in the year ahead.

I lay down on the grass, spread my arms, my legs, remember when I used to make angels in the snow. We lived on Eightieth Street then, and my mother did crossword puzzles every day. My mother. Have I forgiven her? I say I have, but have I really? I am still so cynical about the idea of creating a family. To me the word *family* is synonymous with chaos and pain.

My mother tells this story: *When I married your father, we were poor. He was working as a pants folder in Alexander's department store. We decided he should go to law school at night, and since he was going to be gone all day and then again at night, he asked me what he could do to make the loneliness better. I told him I wanted two things: a television set and a baby. He bought me the TV, and nine months later you were born.*

This is what I remember: a spindly birthday candle with blue and pink paint, a shiny white high chair, a room with a scary mask made out of coconut shell.

You were my best friend. I was alone in New York by then. My grandmother had died, my sister had run away to New Orleans, and Nana and Bepa had moved to Texas. You were my only family, you and Dad, but he was never home. He brought you into our bed as soon as he left in the morning. We would go back to sleep, and when we woke up, we would cuddle and play. You were such a happy, giggly baby. I called you "My Merry Sunshine."

A smell like burning leaves in autumn, another smell like ripples of midnight blue, my father throwing me in the air, a silver medallion hanging on his chest, sitting on my mother's lap at the ocean's edge and being afraid that the rushing water would pull me away from her. The luscious feeling of her. Of Mother.

I didn't really know your dad when we got married. All the other boys thought I was too fat, but your dad thought I was pretty. I'd been going out with him a few weeks when my parents decided to move to Texas, and my mother told me I could either move with them or marry your father, but either way they weren't going to pay for college anymore. I dropped out of school—I was in my first year—and married your dad.

By the time your brother was born, your father had

graduated from law school. We went on our first vacation, and I realized I didn't love him. I felt trapped, I wanted out of the marriage, but my mother got down on her hands and knees and begged me not to divorce him. "For the sake of the children," she said. So I didn't. But things changed after that.

For one, I got thin. Finally. My father was standing at the elevator with me the day we left the hospital with your newborn brother, and as we were getting on, he looked at my rear end and said, "Now are you going to lose weight, Ruthie, now?" I was so ashamed of myself. (It never occurred to me to get angry with him for looking at my ass; we didn't get angry with our parents in those days.) As the elevator reached the lobby, I decided that I was going to lose weight, and that was that.

Another thing that changed was that we hired Ann to take care of you and Howard, and I started going out with friends to bars. I met men who told me I was beautiful. I got attention I'd wanted for years.

I had my first affair when you were twelve. After that there was often another man besides your father.

I gained a brother, whom I didn't ask for, didn't want, and lost a mother. Going to her was like walking into a wall. She was there but not there, always impatient, always bored, always waiting to get away. Resentment radiated from her like hot rain sizzles from a sidewalk.

This much I knew when I was four: She didn't want to be where she was. She was young and glamorous, with long painted nails, high slashes of cheekbones, and she wanted the thieves who had stolen her life—the children who ripped at her heart, the husband she didn't love—to give it back.

This much I knew when I was twenty: I was never going to be in the same position as my mother. I was never going to be trapped by children, a husband. Children tied your hands behind your back, were concrete boats attached to your feet. Children stopped you from living your life, from *having* a life. A husband built the cage you lived in with the children—and then he walked out with the keys in his pocket.

It seemed to me that my father had the power, the money, the keys to the cage, and I identified with him. With his humor and his ambition. With his success and his sexism. He pushed me, criticized me, showered me with affection, withdrew his love when I didn't do well in school. If I came home with a report card of all A's and a B, he would study it for a few minutes, take off his glasses, and say, "What happened with the B?"

My father wanted his firstborn to be a son, and when I arrived, he didn't talk to my mother for three days. But then, the story goes, he fell in love with the toothless grin and the baby smells of pink skin mingled with powder and sleep and stars. He ran to my room when he came home at night. "Before he kissed me hello," my mother says, "he would come and see you." By the time my brother was born, my father didn't need a son to fulfill his dreams. I looked exactly like him, had his eyes, his mouth, his nose, the shape of his face; I was on my way to being the son he always wanted.

When I dropped my Phi Beta Kappa key in his hand, I said to myself, "This was for you, Dad. The rest I do for me." It's not true, though. I am still trying to get that last A, still determined to not be my mother.

Or any mother.

> *We evade that which is Eternal when we evade ourselves; for our failures of truth, we ask clear vision:*
> *For those times I turned a deaf ear on the cries of children;*
> *And for those times I turned a deaf ear to the small child within me.*
> *For those times when I believed that I was alone, and that there was no point in reaching out to others;*
> *And for those times when I believed that my temporary helplessness was permanent.*
> *In recalling this pain, I experience it, I heal it, and I commit myself to replacing it with joy in the coming year.*

Matt is quiet, leaning on the tree with his eyes closed. An unbroken spiderweb is hung between two branches of the tree; a horned lark sings. This inner-child thing is beginning to feel old and overused. I wouldn't mind if it was seen as a stepping-stone to healing, if people believed that, at some point, their inner children would get integrated into the adults they are. The idea that we will always have a part that is our inner child, and that this child will never grow up, is contrary to growth and transformation. It glorifies the act of hanging on to wounds forever.

On the other hand, it is impossible to integrate something we deny, and since so much of who we are is locked up in our past, getting in touch with the part of us that is terrified of growing up is a step that can't be skipped or transcended.

The image of Sophia, standing in the last workshop I led, is clear in my mind. She is saying that during the fat-thin fantasy, the one in which you stand before your mother and your father and see yourself fat, then thin, she understood that she needed to stay fat to be close to her mother. She is crying so hard that she is gulping for air.

"I don't want to lose my mother," she says, "but I don't want to be fat for the rest of my life, either."

She describes her mother: two hundred twenty pounds, unhappy with her relationship to Sophia's step-father, no work of her own, an estranged son who lives across the country. Sophia is her best friend; they eat together, they binge together, they commiserate about being fat together.

"I don't want to leave her behind," Sophia says. "If I lose weight, then how will she feel about herself? How will she feel about me?

"The hardest part," she continues through her tears, "is that I am passing this on to my six-year-old daughter. She already covers her plate with a napkin to stop me from eating what she's left. She hears me tell her to eat carrots and then watches me eat oatmeal cookies and potato chips for dinner. In an effort not to lose my mother, I feel like I am losing my daughter."

I tell her that I understand the bind she is in. When

your main connection with someone is through suffering, it's very difficult to change the terms of the contract. You don't know what you are going to lose. And if that person is your mother, and your identity and your self-worth were formed in this relationship, the specter of loss feels unbearable.

Someone else stands, joins Sophia, says that she feels that the main way women keep themselves small is by keeping themselves big. Three hundred and fifty women nod their heads yes, yes, we keep ourselves small by keeping ourselves big.

I ask the group: How else do you keep yourselves small?

They say:

By eating until we are miserable.

By focusing our lives on food and weight.

By sharing our failures, not our successes.

By complaining when we feel like exalting.

By feeling as if people will be threatened by our happiness.

By maintaining the same kind of relationship with ourselves as we had with our mothers.

By feeling as if we cannot go beyond our mothers' lives.

By believing that we are not allowed to have more than they had.

I am four and my mother's pain is a diesel truck lodged on my chest. I want to make her happy, but I don't know what to do. She doesn't like my father. When I am with her, I pretend that I don't like my father either. I hide the gifts he gives me, the chocolate heart, the miniature Japanese doll. I long for time with him—it is the only time I am happy—but I feel so bad that he makes me happy and makes her miserable. I want to suffer with my mother, so I learn to be depressed. I also learn to agree with the way she sees me (asking for too much, selfish, noisy); then, at least, we are on the same side.

I am twenty-three and I am visiting my maternal grandmother in San Antonio. She is talking about how proud she is of my mother because she is thin. She is saying that my mother looks beautiful and has everything a woman could ask for: a husband and two children. "She doesn't have work," I say. "She doesn't realize how talented she is. She doesn't have a focus for her energy." "Work," my grandmother says, "who needs it? The world revolves on a stiff cock, not on women's work."

I am thirty, and my mother and I are on the phone. When are you going to stop running around the country and settle down, get married, have children? she asks. "Children? Why would I want to have children?" "Children are life's biggest blessing," she says. "Nothing you do will ever come close to bringing you the joy that children bring." "Your life wasn't so joyful, Mom," I say.

I am forty-three and my friend Meredith reads the first draft of this book. She says, "The person you portray in the book is a person who suffers constantly. You don't round yourself out, you don't show the fullness of your life. Why not?"

Because it's not nice. Because people don't like people who brag. Because if I have enough, it means that someone else doesn't, and so it's wrong to have enough.

"I don't want to lose my mother," Sophia says again.

I nod. I don't want to lose my mother, either.

But the truth is, you can't lose anyone who is already lost. I lost my mother when she decided that she would make up for her lost years rather than be a mother. Sophia lost her mother in a sea of food and lovelessness; when her mother chose to eat rather than to feel, there was nothing Sophia could do. We lose our mothers when they are lost to themselves, and there is nothing we can do.

You can't find someone who wants to be lost. You can't find someone until they find themselves. At best, you can diminish your own vitality and swim with them in mutual misery. Most of us chose (and continue to choose) this way of relating, and we call this being alive: diminishing ourselves so that we don't lose someone we never had; keeping ourselves small so that no one is threatened; turning to food the very minute we feel happy so that we can feel bad again; finding something wrong in everything that is right; lying to our friends by not sharing the immensity of the joys and victories; feeling threatened by other women's successes.

I ask the women in the workshop: What is right about feeling small?

What would be shaken up and what would be lost if we allowed ourselves to have big lives?

Why is an embarrassment of riches embarrassing?

We deny that which is Eternal when we deny our own depths.

For the misdeeds we have committed with our bodies and souls, we here today seek to speak them out, expose them to the air, to our tears, to our laughter.

For not being present in the moment, and instead, being off somewhere else, worrying;

For not allowing ourselves to play;

For focusing only on our shortcomings, and not on our strengths and beauties . . .

Why do I feel as if I am *not allowed* to have a big life?

I loved my mother more than anything in the world. She was a golden apparition of blond hair, silky clothes and flowery smells, and I would have done anything for her—taking away my own happiness was a small act compared to the love I felt, the longing to wrap my soul around hers. As a four-year-old, being depressed was an act of compassion for a parent who was miserable. As a forty-three-year-old, being depressed is a habit that I've honed into a skill.

I notice that when I talk to my mother, still, I talk about what is wrong. I talk about feeling fat or confused or tired. I notice, too, that when I talk to friends, I talk about my uncertainties, not my victories, my pain, not my joy. It would never occur to me to say, "I had such a satisfying writing day." Instead I say, "I didn't get much sleep last night, and writing under a deadline is grueling." It's not that the last statement isn't true, it's just that it's not the whole truth, or even the main truth. It's a part of the truth, a tributary of a roaring river. But roaring is not feminine or becoming or humble.

What does this have to do with having a baby?

Having a baby means that I have to stop being a baby, which means that I have to stop being a child who is frightened of losing her mother.

If I am unwilling to lose her, then I continue to believe that I am exactly like her. I feel trapped by anything or anyone that needs something from me. Identifying with her means living with a gnawing in my heart, believing that something better is around the next corner, and whatever I have now is not enough.

There is no better way to be close to my mother than to feel as if I *am* her. That she is me and I am her, and if I have a child, I will feel like a caged, hunted animal, and I will pace, and I will do the same thing to my daughter that my mother did to me. Having a child means being disloyal to my mother's pain at mothering. It means believing that it could be different for me.

For the blessings I lost by not trusting myself;
And for the blessings I lost by not trusting others;
For withholding love and support;
And for being judgmental of others and myself.

For *thinking I would run out of love if I gave too much of it away;*

And *for doubting my ability to love and receive love from others.*

It is one o'clock, and I am very hungry and just as cranky. I begin telling myself that people who have been sick for three years are not expected to fast on Yom Kippur, that fasting will probably make me terribly ill, I might go into a hypoglycemic attack, and Matt will have to rush me off the island to a hospital. God will understand if I eat, I say to myself, as a piece of cinnamon toast with almond butter and bananas floats into my consciousness.

We brush ourselves off and begin walking through a densely wooded grove of fir trees, logs covered with jewel green moss, small acorn-colored chipmunks whose tails bob up, down, sideways each time they chirp at us for disturbing them. When we get to a clearing, I tell Matt I want to sit down, my legs are woozy. We had planned a four-mile walk on a trail that edges the side of the mountain, dips through enchanted, sun-dappled forest, and ends with views of Puget Sound, Mount Baker, the Cascades. At this moment, though, the snow-covered mountains look like vanilla ice cream cones and the clouds like mashed potatoes. Thoughts of being holy have leaked from my body, and I am so hungry that I am on the verge of raving, so I decide to sit down and breathe. Remember that people without homes, without food, feel this way every single day. Remember that millions of Jews are probably feeling the same way at this very moment. (Or else they are in Israel, where it is ten hours ahead, and they are breaking their fast with apples and honey, sweet potatoes and roast chicken. Challah with thick smears of butter . . .)

Matt says, "We don't have to go any farther than this. Let's just sit and look at the mountains, watch the birds. Maybe the eagles are back." We find a large rock with a flat ledge. Around the next bend, past a lily pond and a meadow of swaying grass, is where Matt asked me to marry him five years ago.

My stomach is rumbling, rocking. I look at my husband; he is searching the sky for eagles.

If there are any cages in this marriage, it is I who have built them. And I who hold the key to their locks.

Matt is a meandering walk through the country; I am a labryinth with false starts and mirrored corridors. He is easy and wakes up laughing; I am intense and have never woken up laughing in my life. Our marriage is a quilt of extremes. We fight about his optimism (which I call denial), my introspection (which he calls wallowing). And we struggle with issues of time, money, sex, friends, work. But ours is not my parents' marriage, and I am not my mother.

This hunger is poignant inside my body, a counterpoint to the food I ate last night, to the food I will eat tonight, to the overflowing abundance of my life. To the fact that I am not on the streets, begging for my next meal. This hunger is real hunger, a counterpoint to the phantom hunger of never having or being enough. Of my endless search for B's amidst a cornucopia of A's.

I could spend the rest of my life digging for B's, the way an archaeologist digs for bones. The way I used to hunt for Ninas.

On Sunday mornings my father handed us the Hirschfeld cartoon in the Arts and Leisure section of the *New York Times*, and my brother and I would scramble to see who could find the most Ninas. Nina was the name of Hirschfeld's daughter, and attached to his signature, in the lower right corner, was the number of times her name appeared in the cartoon. Sometimes the Ninas jumped out at you—they were spiky, part of someone's hair or hem. But more often than not they were so cleverly placed that you couldn't find the last one or two. After a while our eyes would hurt from examining the intricacies of sleeves, collars, fingernails, buckles, and we'd stop. But I never gave up. I kept the drawing on my desk, scouring it a few times a day, and eventually I'd find that last Nina. By that time it was Tuesday and no one cared. They were busy with the rest of their lives.

No one whom I care about cares about the B's. My father has long put down his glasses, and Matt is searching for eagles. I could keep hunting for the ways I don't measure up. I could stay immobilized by the ways I am like my mother, or I could realize that Sunday has passed, it's Tuesday now, and time to live the rest of my life.

The mountains won't crash and the sky won't turn black and God won't punish me if I feel good, feel happy, feel pleasure. Suffering is not admirable. Pain is not noble. Tearing myself down will not help me build myself up.

Pain is only worth what it takes you to; it is not meant to be a way of life.

I've used it as a defense:

If I know how damaged I am, then I won't be hurt when you don't love me.

If I take happiness away from myself, then you can't take it from me.

If I keep myself from loving you completely, then I won't be devastated when I get a phone call in the middle of the night telling me you are dead.

If I don't have children, then I can't be a terrible mother.

It's not pain I am frightened of; it's joy. But it's Tuesday now, and the second half of my life stretches before me. It is time to take a risk.

I don't need to be faithful to my mother's pain anymore. If she does not have enough, despite the riches in her life, I am still allowed to be wildly, exuberantly happy with what I have. If having children tied concrete boats to her feet, they might still wrap gossamer wings on mine.

I have a choice.

I will not break if Matt dies, but I will break if he dies and I held myself back from loving him. The pain of being criticized for my books is nothing compared to the agony I would feel if I didn't write them. And the only thing more frightening than taking the leap and having children, or taking the leap into anything you are frightened of, is not taking the leap. To get to the end of your life and say, "I lived unknown to myself"—that is the biggest risk.

And again, I remember:
my non-involvement;
failing to love;
failing to see the humor.

Keep reminding me that the Talmud says I will be called to account for all the permitted pleasures I failed to enjoy.

On this day of Yom Kippur, in the Jewish new year of 5755, I ask to be forgiven for turning my back on the A's of my life, the daily joys of being with Matt, the pleasure of making words into a book. The ice-cream mountains, the jewel green moss. The growl of hunger in my stomach. My body that has not given up, despite the years of hard-boiled eggs and spinach diets.

In naming these lost blessings, I let go of regret and bitterness, I recognize the inexhaustibility of life's blessings, and I vow to be open to these blessings as they come to me in this coming year.

I send out a prayer to God, to the mountains, to the eagles, to the earth: If there is a spirit who knows who I am and still wants me for a mother, you are a tough little being, and I'm here, waiting, with arms flung open and gossamer wings at my feet.

Chapter Seven

■

PARALLEL LIVES,
PART 2:
ON HAPPINESS
AND JOY

■

M att and I arrive at the acupuncturist's office on Tenth and Tenth in Oakland. He settles himself on a torn vinyl chair; I take one with fat red cushions and pick up a book on the table called *Natural Healing for Pets*. In the chapter on communication, the author writes that it is possible to converse with your dog or cat. "You can," she says, "ask them questions like 'How about ice cream for dinner?' Or 'Where did you come from before you showed up at the animal shelter?' If you quiet your mind and send visual images, they will send images back."

I imagine sending images to Blanche, our cat. I'd ask him what he thinks about all day, and he'd send me a picture of a large tuna fish. "Listen to this," I say to Matt, but the door opens and Dr. Rudolph walks in.

She is wearing a teal blue shirt with yellow submarines printed on it. Her hair has been cut short; it stands in spikes on the top of her head. "So, how's the patient today?" she asks.

"A little grumpy," I answer.

She peers in the Kennel Cab. "Mr. Blanche?"

Matt and I walk to the table on which the carrier is perched. I open the grated door. "C'mon, Blanche. Time to come out and see Dr. Rudolph." He glowers at me. I send him a visual image of walking out of the box. He hunkers down in the back, folds his paws beneath his chest. Glares. I send another image.

"Geneen!" Matt says. "What are you staring at him for? Grab the back of the box and help me pull him out."

"I was trying to talk to him in visual images," I say as I turn the carrier upside down, gravity being the only force strong enough to move Blanche onto the table.

Matt ignores the comment. As I hold the carrier, he pulls Blanche. Yanks his two front paws out of the box. The rest of his twenty-pound body appears reluctantly. Sasha, my nine-year-old friend, says Blanche looks like a cloud "because he's white and big and goes on forever." Matt's friend Gregory says that he looks like a lamb because the fur on his chest is curly. I think he looks like the toy cat my mother gave me when I was eight; it was white and silky with blue eyes and a red ribbon. But whereas the toy cat had porcelain eyes and a wispy tail, Blanche has eyes that are crossed and a tail that's as bushy as pampas grass. And whereas the toy cat fit snugly in the crook of my arm, Blanche, when splayed on the quilt, takes up a third of the bed. If he sleeps on— not under or in the crook of—my arm, I have to spend the next ten minutes waving it around, coaxing the blood to circulate. Blanche is not the kind of cat anyone—friends, plumbers, delivery people—can ignore; when he stalks into a room, you stop what you are doing and stare.

Blanche is an event.

A few years ago, I wanted to change his name to Butterfly, but my mother pointed out that he looked more like a moose than a butterfly, and anyway (she said), wouldn't it confuse him to have his name changed after seven years? Wasn't it bad enough that Blanche was a girl's name and he was a boy?

Dr. Rudolph says, "Let me look at you, Blanche." He turns his back to us, faces the wall, and flips his tail twice. "Happy to see me as usual," she says, taking his jaw in her hands and opening his mouth to check his teeth. Next, she uses her stethoscope to listen to his heart, asks us questions about his energy, appetite. She begins putting needles in a row on each side of his spine.

"Hey," Matt says, "how did that conference go? Did you play the saxophone for your audience?" The last time we were here, she was preparing a speech for a Midwest veterinary conference. Matt encouraged her to play her saxophone as part of the talk, and to have the audience meow and bark.

"No, but I did ask them to make the sounds their animals made—they loved it, all that howling and meowing and barking."

Blanche growls, yaps, growls again. "It's the liver point," she says, "it's stagnant."

"The liver point always seems to be stagnant," I say. "Why?"

She raises her eyebrows and points at his generously proportioned physique. "It's his *size*, Geneen, his size."

Ah, his size.

It *is* true that Blanche is very large, although we recently heard that the *Guinness Book of World Records* lists the largest cat as forty-three pounds. And my editor once sent me an article from the *National Enquirer* about a seventy-five-pound cat who terrorized and then ate two chihuahuas.

It is also true that when people first see Blanche, they usually say, "Oh my God, what *is* that? It can't be a cat . . ." or "That is the biggest thing I've ever seen." Matt, offended, will often counter with "Big? Compared to what? Blanche is *small* compared to most animals . . ." Then he'll bend down and rub Blanche's ears to demonstrate how small Blanche is compared to a horse, for instance. Or a cow.

After visitors finish exclaiming about Blanche's size, they start carrying on about what he can do about it. "Hey, Geneen, how come you don't give Blanche one of your books to read, hah hah hah?" And inevitably, "Have you ever thought about leading compulsive eating groups for cats, hah hah hah?" Everyone thinks they are the first to make the connection between my books and my cat.

Last week my cousin Lily was visiting and she said, "How is it that you ended up with the fattest cat in the universe? There are no accidents, you know. Blanche is fat because you are thin . . ."

I thought of my friend Sabrina, who told me that when she was growing up and going on diets, she made her brother eat everything she wasn't allowed. If she wanted a piece of cheesecake, she bribed him into sitting at the table while she ate cottage cheese and he ate cheesecake. He spent weeks wolfing down Oreos and Mallomars while she ate tomatoes and dry toast. When she wanted a chocolate malted, which he drank, and then demanded that he eat a liverwurst and pimento sandwich with mayonnaise, ketchup, and sweet pickles, he ended the game.

But as far as I know, I didn't do that with Blanche. Of course, it is possible that I did it unconsciously, since unconsciousness and food go together in my psyche like cream cheese and jelly. I have relived his kittenhood, racked my brain for hidden intentions, for passive-aggressive behaviors. I ask myself if this is a case of "cat acts out mother's shadow," but the truth is, I can't figure out how he got this big. This, er, fat.

Okay, so I might have overdone it on the baby food and dried sardines, but that was nine years ago. He was a sickly kitten, always getting colds, fevers, refusing to eat, and he *liked* baby food. How could I refuse him? And it is possible that the sprouted rye bread, butternut squash, sweet potatoes, corn, mashed potatoes, tuna fish, chicken, and cantaloupe I give him don't help him lose weight, but at a nibble here, a smidgen there, he probably uses more calories by chewing the food than he gets from eating it.

Besides, Blanche is not compulsive about food. If anything, he is a delicate and discriminating eater. Last night Matt was trying to teach him to eat corn on the cob. He couldn't get the right amount of tension in his paws to hold the cob, so Matt ended up biting off five or six kernels at a time and letting Blanche eat them out of his hand. After a few rounds Blanche turned on his paws and walked into the living room: he'd had enough. He eats when he's hungry, stops when he's full, skips meals when he is frightened, excited, anxious, sick, lonely. When you eat that way, you reach your natural weight. The only conclusion that makes any sense is that this *is* Blanche's natural weight, and it happens to be significant.

When I tell this to my friend Sally, who foisted Blanche on me because she said it was time for me to have a cat, and kept his only living relatives—his sister and mother—she points out that he comes from stock that is lean and lithe, six and seven pounds respectively. She points out that she has never thrown out a vertebrae by picking up *her* cats, so perhaps I should reconsider this natural-weight theory. I point out that girl cats are smaller than boy cats, and that most luminaries are different from the rest of their families. Take Einstein, for instance. Or Arnold Schwarzenegger.

I watch Blanche carefully for any signs of self-consciousness about his size. The fact that we have to go shopping for his carrier in the Big Animals Department of the pet store. The fact that when he comes through his cat door, there is always a moment of uncertainty, when his paws and his head have gotten through, but the rest of him, the base of the pyramid, is still on the other side. He hesitates. I hold my breath. And then he manages to lift his legs, push through the plastic flap, and appear in the house. I clap, exclaim that he is brilliant, agile, a wonder among cats. Blanche looks at me, disgusted, as if to say, "Haven't you got anything better to do? Aren't you supposed to be writing a book?"

He is shameless. About his needs, his foibles. His size. Once he fell in the hot tub because he made a running jump for the ledge and overshot his target. Allowing himself to be retrieved, he shook himself off, looked pityingly at me (and Sally, who was crying from laughing so hard) because we were still stuck in a vat of hot water, and walked delicately onto the deck.

He doesn't let his weight stop him from climbing trees, squeezing into paper lunch bags, sleeping in drawers half his size. From asking for attention, affection, and, if he doesn't get it, demanding it—by walking on the computer keyboard and putting his weight on the letter A, by settling on my chest when I am sleeping and placing his paw on my face.

Since I read that book in Dr. Rudolph's office, I have been trying to send images to Blanche. The author said that when you are leaving, say, for three days, you should look at your cat and imagine the passing of three days, three nights, so that he will know when you will be back.

I do that, but I feel as if I am speaking someone else's language, not Blanche's and mine.

We already talk to each other. Not in discrete images, but in flashes of feeling, facial expressions, unspoken intentions. If it is possible to know an animal who is still part wild, to penetrate the mystery of any being, I know this animal. I sense him before I see him, know what he wants before he asks. Because no words pass between us, the communication takes place along ribbons of feeling that flutter from him to me to him throughout the house, throughout the day.

Storytellers say that everyone has a soul animal. Witches have "familiars," their power animals; I have Blanche. He couldn't have been other than he is, couldn't have been sleek or lean. Then he would have fit my idea of what my cat was supposed to look like, of what I am supposed to look like; then he wouldn't have cracked the lichee nut of my heart.

His size was the wild card; he is so startling in his bigness, such a contrast to the obsession with thinness that has run my life. And because he defies all my images of size, because his weight is a given to him, a fact, because there is no angsting, no wobbling, no wishing to be any different, he is a constant reminder of life beyond appearances. Of the dignity and sensuality that is our birthright, regardless of size: lapping up a splash of sun, being stroked exactly where and for how long you like it, playing for the joy of it. And although I know that he is a cat and I am a person, his unbroken connection to spirit and

instinct is like sweet summer rain on the parched river-
bed of mine.

Recently, a friend told me about Dr. Marcy Meyer, a
Ph.D. clinical psychologist who is "an animal communicator" via the telephone. When you call her (in New
York, by the way, not California), you tell her your animal's name, physique, date of birth, and topics you want
her to discuss with your pet. If, for instance, your dog is
sick, you tell this to Marcy, along with any questions you
have about how long the illness will last, what your dog
needs from you as well as what the dog is trying to teach
you. My friend Rianne, who told me about the communicator, explained that her friend with a dying dog
named Tofu was told by Marcy, who was told by Tofu,
that the dog had taken on cancer to prevent her friend
from getting it. Tofu said that she had lived a long and
happy life and that she was not afraid of dying. Tofu also
told Marcy when she would die—and according to
Rianne's friend, that's exactly when she did.

"Why are you telling me this?" I asked suspiciously.

"I thought you might want to speak to Blanche
through Marcy."

Every one of my friends knows I am a sucker when it
comes to Blanche. A pushover, a believer, a wimp. For
my birthday last year, Matt made a videotape of Blanche,
complete with special effects, spins, fade-ins, fade-outs.
He went to a studio in San Francisco, where he rented a
high-tech machine that could edit hours of Blanche (at
the acupuncturist's, drinking water, playing, walking,

wearing his red fez) into a three-and-a-half-minute video, while "Doo Wah Ditty" played in the background.

I asked Rianne what she thought Blanche would want to say to me. "What else? He'd talk to you about his size, Geneen," she said, "and the connection with your work."

That evening I tell Matt about Dr. Marcy Meyer, and he looks at me as if I've lost my mind. He says that it was bad enough when I wanted to take Blanche to the cat chiropractor, but this is going too far. In so many words, and with a great deal of compassion, he tells me to get a life.

Undaunted, I mention that Dr. Nelson, the cat chiropractor, *helped* Blanche—he stopped limping after the neck adjustment—and anyway, who knows what's true or what's possible? No one thought the earth was round. What about the scientists who talk with dolphins? And Koko, the gorilla, who speaks in sign language?

During the next few weeks I find myself wondering what I would ask Blanche if I could really speak to him. What he would say to me if he could really answer. It's not his size per se that interests me; it's his unconditional acceptance of his size. It's the fact that he is who he is and he doesn't seem to spend his life wanting to be a sleeker cat. Or a dachshund.

Stephen Levine, a meditation teacher, says that hell is not fire and brimstone, not a place where you are punished for lying or cheating or stealing. Hell is wanting to be something and somewhere different from where you are.

If that is true, and I believe it is, most of us spend most of our lives in hell.

In one of my life's least fine and thoroughly hypocritical moments, I decided that I was going to look like Madonna. It wasn't her face or her hair I wanted. It wasn't even her body as a unit. I wanted her arms. I wanted her biceps. To look like a photograph I'd seen of her wearing a sleeveless black dress and extending her arms, biceps glistening, announcing her strength.

I'd wanted muscles for years. I wanted to prove to myself (to the ghosts in my head, the boys in my elementary school, my ninth-grade English teacher, and everyone who had ever made fun of me in my life) that even I, a.k.a. Cottage Cheese Thighs and Chicken Wing Arms, could be sleek, taut, muscular. I wanted revenge the way a child wants it, the way she imagines everyone who has ever hurt her weeping at her funeral. And somehow I convinced myself (this took a lot of convincing, since my life's work is about what women do to themselves in the name of being thin, and *When Food Is Love* was soon to be published) that building muscles was an important way to spend my time, and that I would feel immensely gratified by setting a goal and meeting it. I convinced myself that having biceps would change something fundamental about my life. That changing my body would change my psyche. Would unzip the cloud where happiness is stored.

I consulted with a personal trainer. She told me I

needed to cut fat out of my diet (even tofu has too much fat, she told me) and start working out with weights twice a week, increase my aerobic workouts to six days a week, sixty minutes a session. I welcomed the challenge, stopped using butter, olive oil, stopped eating anything with fat. I lost weight, developed small but noticeable muscles on my arms.

My images of touring with *When Food Is Love*, being on national television and showing my muscles to the American public, were squashed when the book was published in February, and blizzards across the country necessitated wearing long underwear at all times.

In New York City for the tour, I was in a cab with my publicist. We had spent the hour between interviews shopping, and she was commenting on how sleek and lean I looked. I thought about it for a moment and said, "The problem is that I have to work so hard for this body that it doesn't feel like mine."

When I worked out every day, I was preparing for a life that I was never going to lead. I was lifting barbells so that I could dance on stage with bare arms and bare legs, so that I could wear strapless dresses at fabulous events, so that I could go on television in clothes that are more appropriate for a stripper than a writer. I wanted to have muscles so that I could fulfill yet another requirement of my parallel life, my fantasy world. If I had the right body, I would have the right life.

I am not dismissing working hard. Writing books, teaching workshops, maintaining relationships, all take hard work. But while I am doing them, I am present, I am totally engaged in and passionate about the process. I am not tapping my foot, watching the clock, waiting to be excused.

Some women enjoy lifting weights.

I am not one of them.

But neither am I dismissing exercise. Most afternoons, after a day of writing, I put on a sweatsuit and go hiking. I hike because I need to use my body after so many hours of using my mind, because I want to be among trees, because I love to sweat, work my legs, swing my arms. Because it clears my mind and cleans my body. I do not hike to develop quadriceps. The body I develop from hiking is incidental to the sensuality and pleasure of the activity itself.

My friend Carolyn says she is exhilarated by lifting weights; it makes her feel strong and capable in the rest of her life. I say, good, keep doing what exhilarates you, but do it *because* it exhilarates you, not because it will bring you something you think you need to have to be acceptable, to be allowed to live your life.

A Berkeley performance artist named Nina Wise tells a story that was told to her by Carlos Castaneda, author of the Don Juan books. Castaneda, under an alias, spent a year working in a greasy-spoon restaurant in Tucson, during which time his closest friend was a waitress named Linda. Without knowing that he was the man who wrote them, she gave Castaneda the Don Juan books to read, saying that she was a big fan of his. One day a white limousine pulled up in back of the restaurant, and someone told Linda that Castaneda was inside. She wanted desperately to meet him, but told her best friend (Castaneda himself) that she was too fat, and was certain that the famous author would ignore her. After the man she thought was Castaneda spurned her, the real Castaneda comforted Linda as she cried in his arms. The real Castaneda thought Linda was beautiful and radiant.

She never discovered that she was loved and admired by the man whose love and admiration she was hungering for. She didn't need to lose weight, change her hair, go to a workshop; she already was who she imagined she needed to be.

We construct parallel lives based on what we think will make us feel worthy, beautiful, loved, while the real thing, our lives as they are, spread before us, unused, unsung. We become so convinced we have to look, think, feel, act in ways that match our parallel lives, we miss the moment-to-moment unfolding that could, at last, satisfy us.

A parallel life—our fantasy of what will happen when we turn a final corner and find the love, respect, visibility, and abundance that's eluded us for a lifetime—is the adult version of the childhood longing to be seen and loved. When as children we understand that we are not going to get that love, we make up stories, create a fantasy life, try to be someone else. And when we believe that love will be waiting around the corner if only we could transform ourselves into different people, we will spend our lives trying to turn that corner.

But there are many obstacles in trying to be someone else.

The first is that it's impossible. You cannot be someone else. Period. The second obstacle is that no matter how hard you try, and no matter how many wonderful, kind, sensitive, politically correct, and altruistic acts you perform, it is never enough. You have to keep doing more and more to silence the part of you that knows your actions are based on fear of what would happen if you didn't try so hard. The you that you believe yourself to be is always lurking in the shadow of the you that is trying to be loved.

The third obstacle is that you never allow yourself to feel the original hopelessness of knowing there was nothing you could do in your family to be loved or seen or honored. As a child that kind of despair is too frightening, too immense to feel, so you protect yourself from it by developing elaborate defense mechanisms, i.e., believing that you can fix what is wrong by changing who you are. As an adult you no longer need those defenses, yet they have become so habitual that you accept them as "the way you are." You think of them as efforts to improve yourself.

But it takes a lot of activity not to feel the way you feel, and so your life is lived between frantic extremes. When you are not trying as hard as you can to be your idea of a worthy person, when you are not eating correctly and being nice and giving away all your time, you binge on everything in sight, and you feel selfish and angry and mean-spirited. You are either squeezing yourself into a narrow, tight version of acceptable behavior, or you are crashing through the tightness and rebelling against everything that constricts you. Both are defenses against feeling the original hopelessness; the main purpose of these defenses is to keep you safe by engaging in a war that is besides the point. The main problem with these defenses is that you forget they are defenses. You begin to believe them.

Take, for instance, the war with food and your body.

You swing from dieting to bingeing, from being thin to being fat, and everyone thinks you have an eating problem. *You* think you have an eating problem, but you don't.

The problem is not with food because even if you get thin and stay thin for fifty years, if you don't work with the root of the struggle, you will always feel as if your happiness lies around the next corner, the next accomplishment. You will be thin, but you will still be afraid of getting fat, and you will still spend your life swinging from one extreme to the next. You will never know who you are, and you will never leave yourself alone.

The real work of this life is not what we do every day from nine to five. The real work is to disidentify from self-images that were formed a lifetime ago, and from which we still construct our daily lives. The real work is to allow ourselves to be who we already are, and to have what we already have. The real work is to be passionate, be holy, be wild, be irreverent, to laugh and cry until you awaken the sleeping spirits, until the ground of your being cleaves and the universe comes flooding in.

How do we do that work? How do we dream our own lives into being when we've spent those lives wanting to be different than we are?

By understanding that the more time we spend constructing parallel lives, the less energy we have for our present lives.

By respecting the valid reasons we create those lives: the need to be seen, recognized, and honored for our deepest, truest selves.

By allowing ourselves to feel, millimeter by millimeter and only with support, the original hopelessness that so much of our frantic activity covers up.

By constantly inquiring into our experience: Does getting what we want take away the discomfort of wanting, or is one longing replaced by another and then another?

By honoring the longing to have a big life, which can either translate into the longing to have someone else's life or the longing to have the life you would already have if you were not constantly diminishing yourself.

By having role models besides models or actresses.

By realizing that having role models who are leaders or healers or scientists or artists or mothers is not the answer, either. Role models are examples of women who are inhabiting *their* lives; our work is to discover, and then inhabit, our own lives.

By living daily with the burning question that is behind every addiction: What is enough?

By understanding that our lives unfold as we live with, and burn with, our questions. There is no right answer. By knowing that no feeling is final.

By stopping ourselves each time we notice that we are evaluating ourselves against another person's accomplishments. Comparisons are self-defeating, exhausting, and deadly.

By seeing that everyone is in the process of becoming and that no one, no matter how much love or beauty or money she has, is more or less perfect than we are. Every single person is wounded, just as everyone has a right to speak, to take up space, to live a big, magnificent life.

By being aware that what you do to get somewhere is who you become when you arrive. The process is the goal. You cannot spend your life wanting to be someone else, snipping off pieces of yourself you don't like, and suddenly expect, upon reaching a goal, to be confident, self-accepting, rooted like an oak tree in your being.

Thich Nhat Hanh, the Vietnamese Buddhist master, says: "There is no way to happiness; happiness is the way." The only way to increase the size of your life is to live a bigger life now.

It is said that a person dies the way she lives. If her life has been fearful, anxious, tormented, if she always wants to be somewhere else, someone else, her dying will be etched with fear, will bring her no peace. In this same way, our lives become the color of, are nothing more than, each minute, hour, day we live. If we spend our time wanting to be different than we are, we will never be free.

Now, I realize that as a reader, your mind has strayed far from my cat, and that talking about Blanche right now may seem incongruous with the seriousness of the topic, but let me assure you that I know no better example than Blanche of a being who is not tormented by the issues at hand. My friend Janet says that he is her guru because "he is who he is and that's enough."

Blanche knows what his priorities are, and trying to be different is not one of them. He knows that if you can run, feel the wind in your fur, and sit in the leafy shade of trees, the size of your body and the size of your spirit are a true match. To Blanche the same old things— dripping water, ants, ballpoint pens, dust—are new every day; he lives in a perpetual state of acceptance and wonder. When I lost my hair, eyebrows, and eyelashes, his affection for me remained constant. But the question is: Is he unconcerned about my appearance because he doesn't want attention focused on his? Does he accept his body because he doesn't know about the dangers of cholesterol? Is he in denial about his pyramidlike physique, or is he profoundly wise?

This, I decided, was a case for Dr. Marcy Meyer, animal communicator, feline mind melder. With phone in hand, and Blanche splayed on the leopard-print chair beside me, it took Dr. Meyer a few minutes to tune into Blanche's frequency. After five minutes of silence, she told me that Blanche was an old soul and very wise. I asked her how she knew that, hoping that Blanche was not bragging about himself. She said that when you talk to animals all day long, you can tell the old souls from the new souls. "It's the way he contemplates," she said.

I told her that Blanche is a trickster, and that he often looks as if he is contemplating because his eyes are crossed. Then I asked her to ask him about his weight. Blanche mumbled a few words about respecting my body, treating it well, and not worrying so much about food.

"Never mind about *my* body," I said. "Will you please ask him about his body? Why he is so fat?"

Dr. Meyer, clearly exasperated with my focus on the superficial manifestation of Blanche's soul, suggested that I speak to Blanche about contemplation because that was what he wanted to teach me. I told her that I didn't want to know about contemplation, I wanted to know about fat.

The problem was that Blanche did not consider himself fat. When Dr. Meyer asked him about his body size, he said that he doesn't give it much attention and neither should I.

Our thirty-minute appointment was up. Dr. Meyer had to go to the zoo and speak to an elephant who refused to eat. I thanked her, hung up the phone, and turned my attention again to Blanche, who was lying on his back with his paws up in the air, blissfully unaware of my efforts to impose meaning on his size.

Perhaps it's not Blanche that is so unusual, but the fact that I love him completely, without wanting to change him. And since love for a cat is still love, since all love flows from and returns to the same dewy cave in my chest, the possibility exists to greet myself and other two-legged creatures with that same kind of open-ended acceptance, curiosity, and wonder.

My friends with children say it's the quality of love that is so unique, the fact that you surrender yourself to love, and through that surrendering become transparent to your deepest feelings. Perhaps it's not having a child that is so striking, but that unconditional love, joy, happiness exist and finally, through the child, have a chance to be expressed. To finally, irrevocably love without holding anything back. Perhaps the magic—the love, happiness, fulfillment—existed in us all along like an underground river, but we could never see it or know it because we kept looking for it outside, in accomplishments, body sizes, and other people.

Blanche opens his eyes, blinks twice. He stands, stretches his back, jumps off the chair, and waits patiently at the door. When I let him out, he watches a bluejay for the nine hundredth time and acts as if he's never seen a bird before. I notice how happy I am watching him, and notice, too, that it's not a happiness that is about relationship; it doesn't belong to Blanche, or even to Blanche and me. This is a silky gold kind of happiness, a ripple of light that seems to exist through me, with a presence of its own. This is the very same happiness that I thought I would feel if I was thin enough, famous enough, loved enough.

These, then, are Blanche's gifts to me: the knowledge that I am capable of this kind of happiness, and the experience of happiness as something that already exists inside me, rather than something that will finally happen to me when I do or achieve the right combination of things.

Blanche chases the bird, then becomes enraptured by a caterpillar with saffron spots. After a moment he loses interest and walks to a spot of sun, rolls in the dirt. Keeps rolling from one side to the other, basking in the heat, making his fur a comfortable nest for ants, fleas, and leaves. The sun is brassy and hot, the sky a swatch of pale blue. I feel like watermelon tastes: clear, honeyed, endless. A bougainvillea blossom falls and catches in my hair. As I turn to go back in the house and feel the cool, slatted floor beneath my feet, I realize that this is what enough feels like.

Chapter Eight

■

THE LONGING FOR
A SAFE PLACE

■

I suppose you could say that October 17, 1989, was a bad hair day.

Mr. Lee had taken the first snip of my wet hair when the building started to shake. At first I thought a fire truck was barreling down the street. Then I realized it was an earthquake, and I calmed down. Having lived through many earthquakes in fifteen years, I know they follow a predictable pattern: They start, they rattle, they end. In a moment this one would end as well. I watched as bottles of Fuchsia Pink and Passion Red nail polish rolled off the counters; a mirror fell off its hinges and shattered on the floor. Spiky combs in jars filled with cobalt blue disinfectant tipped over and spilled like fans on the slick tile floor.

"It's an earthquake!" shouted a woman with turquoise hair as she ran into the doorway and braced herself against it.

Another woman, half her hair in rollers, started screaming in a florid language I didn't recognize. When she saw the turquoise-haired woman standing in the doorway, she began running for it as well, but couldn't walk more than a step without losing her balance. After falling twice, she got down on her hands and knees and crawled.

Mr. Lee, scissors in one hand, tried to balance himself on the undulating floor. It occurred to me that the earthquake was lasting a long time, and that I should probably make a move to save myself from the next shattering mirror, but all I could do was sit in the swivel chair, stunned. My body felt as if it were wrapped in wet felt; my mind was a blur of thoughts, feelings—each synapse was miles from the next. Should I run for the door, crawl under a counter, run out of the building? I tried to remember why people said to stand in doorways. Disjointed images flashed through my mind: the silver overlay bottles from Russia that had been passed down to me from my great-grandmother; Blanche, his butterscotch tail sticking straight up as he ran through the pampas grass behind the cottage on Alice Street; the space between Matt's two front teeth. I saw Cliff's face in my old apartment on Cayuga Street, purple corduroy curtains with lemon yellow trim framing his head. If there's an earthquake, he said, crawl under your desk. But I wasn't near my desk. I was on the third story of a rickety building in San Francisco, and the floor kept heaving.

I didn't think I was going to die. I didn't think the building would collapse. I didn't think of fires or exploding gas lines or cars being crushed from telephone poles.

I only thought this was the longest earthquake I had ever lived through and wished it would end. Now. I got out of the chair, walked as best I could to the doorway, and waited.

After it was over, in the darkened building—the lights had gone out, the electricity was off—the woman with turquoise hair picked up the nail polish, mopped the disinfectant, and swept the shards of mirror from the floor. I noticed that her nose was pierced and that the plastic watchband on her right arm matched her hair. The woman with the half permanent ran out of the building, forgetting, or else not caring, that tomorrow her hair would look like the Toni home perm girl gone wild.

Like true Californians, Mr. Lee and I took the earthquake in stride and resumed our positions. He picked up his scissors and began cutting my bangs, made hairdresser talk. He asked me where I lived.

Santa Cruz, I said.

Oh, he answered, do you go to the beach often?

Every day, I said.

What about the boardwalk? he asked.

I've been there only once, I answered, watching carefully as he made his mark on my straight, fine hair. I wouldn't have been at Mr. Lee's if my beloved hairdresser had not tried (unsuccessfully) to kill himself with wine, cocaine, and a running motor in a closed garage. It had taken six weeks from the time I first called to get an appointment with Mr. Lee, so I figured that he was either very good or worked one day a week.

A balding man with a mustache and golf balls on his

tie brought a transistor radio from the office across the hall and placed it on the reception desk. "We've just had a report that the Bay Bridge has collapsed," blared the radio. I didn't believe it. Neither did Mr. Lee. "Those newscasters are always exaggerating," he said. "All they care about is getting people to tune into their station." I nodded slightly, afraid to destroy the straight line of the cut. "They'll do anything for a story," I said.

Mr. Lee finished with my hair. My bangs, I noticed, were crooked, but I didn't care. Any traces of energy had leaked from my body long ago, leaving me papery as birch bark in Vermont December. All I could think about was seeing Matt's face, holding him, feeling the warmth of his body. He'd been on a business trip for two weeks, and we were meeting at the Saint Francis Hotel at six-thirty for a tryst and a jasmine bubble bath. A woman in a pinstripe suit with short silver hair and a maroon bow tie showed up for her appointment with Mr. Lee at six, but the electricity had not been restored and it was getting too dark to see. She made another appointment, and as I walked down the stairs, I thought it unfair that she had to wait five more weeks for a haircut.

Using the image of Matt's face to sustain me, I climbed in my car, turned on the engine, and pointed it toward Union Square. None of the traffic lights were working, telephone poles had fallen down, streets were blocked off. When I pulled up to the Saint Francis, a crowd of businessmen in three-piece suits and name tags were standing outside with vacant, startled looks on their faces. They looked like deer, frozen by the glare of headlights on a moony country road. A pair of elderly identical twins, each with bleached blond hair and bright blue eye shadow, red polka-dot dresses, black pillbox hats, and black patent leather shoes stood on the street corner, holding each other, crying.

I tried to get the doorman's attention. I wanted to tell him I was checking in, ask where I should park. He was busy answering questions, talking to one of the businessmen. When he walked over to my window, I asked him about checking in. He said, "There's been an earthquake. You can't check in and there's no place to park." He walked back to the businessmen. I sat in my car, unable to move or think. I stared at the twins. I noticed the short white gloves they were wearing and wondered how I could have missed seeing those gloves a few minutes ago. My mother used to tell me that a lady always wears gloves, white kid gloves with pearl buttons. My mind drifted to a sky blue organdy party dress I had when I was ten. Someone honked. I looked in my mirror. A man with mirrored sunglasses and a blond ponytail was motioning for me to move.

Matt. I had to find Matt.

I looked at my watch. It was six-thirty. Matt's plane had arrived at five-fifteen, so he must be here by now. I left my car in a no-parking zone and walked into the hotel. A few scattered candles and two or three flashlights lit a lobby teeming with confusion. Throngs of people were gathered in groups; some were wandering in small circles; some were standing still, staring at nothing in particular. The air was charred, as if it had been used up long ago. I felt as if I had entered a movie set of an old western and was witnessing the remains of a once elegant hotel. Using the plastic flashlight on my key chain, I weaved through the crowds to the front desk, which was lit by three candles. The woman in front of me was crying. "I need to find my daughter," she said. "I have to find my daughter. She went up in the elevator right before the earthquake. She's only eight years old, and now she's stuck in the elevator. Can't you do something? She must be frightened to death. You have to get her out. Please, can't you get her out? She's only eight years old. I told her I would be right here, waiting for her when she came back."

The man behind the desk, dressed in the gray-and-black-striped Saint Francis uniform, was clearly overwhelmed by the terror of not just this visitor, but all the visitors who had arrived in San Francisco anticipating walks on Fisherman's Wharf, rides on the cable car, chocolate from Ghirardelli Square, and instead discovered that the thin veneer of knowing what the next moment would bring had been destroyed in seven seconds.

He leaned over the desk, squeezing compassion from his wrung-out heart. "I'm sorry, I'm really sorry that your daughter is stuck in the elevator. We are doing everything we can do to help, and as soon as the electricity is restored, you will see her again. She is safe, don't worry."

He looked past her to me. "Can I help you?"

"I'd like to find out if my husband has checked in, and if he hasn't, I'd like to go to our room and wait for him."

"Our computers are down," he said simply. "There is no way to know whether your husband is here or not. If he arrived after the earthquake, he couldn't have gotten to his room because we wouldn't have known what room to give him, and the elevators are not working. He might be in the lobby. Why don't you look for him there?"

"You mean no one can check in? I can't stay here tonight?"

"I'm sorry, but that's right. Nothing can happen until the electricity is restored, and we have no idea when that will be. Can I help you?" he said, looking over my head to the person behind me.

Turning away from the clerk, I stood next to the desk and stared into the lobby. This isn't happening, I thought, it isn't happening. Numb and feeling completely lost, I walked in the darkness, stumbling over stuffed chairs, feet, coffee tables, calling Matt's name. If he arrived on time, he would have come here to meet me. I was certain that I would find him, and by finding him I would find a circle of safety.

"Matt," I called, "Matt, are you here?"

No answer. I walked through the bar, the tea room, the restaurant. Matt, Matt. The darkness was swallowing the sound of his name, and no matter how many times I called, I couldn't will him around the next corner.

Using the back of an $8.43 receipt from the Staff of Life, I wrote: "I drove back to Santa Cruz. I love you. If you can, come home."

I walked to the front of the line at the check-in desk, handed the note to the same man who had waited on me. He was talking to a woman whose seventy-eight-year-old mother needed her heart medication—she, too, was trapped in an elevator. He scribbled Matt's name on an envelope, and I left.

My car was still there. So were the twins, the doorman, the three-piece suits. One movement followed the other. Open car door. Depress clutch. Put car in first gear. Turn steering wheel. Drive. I glanced at the gas tank, noticed that I had less than a quarter of a tank, not enough to get me the seventy-five miles to Santa Cruz. I remembered what I'd heard about gas stations closing after earthquakes because of ruptures in the gas lines, possible fires. I realized I might have to spend the night, perhaps a few nights, on the side of the road, until electricity was restored and motels could open and gas stations could start pumping gas. I didn't have any water, I didn't have any food, a fever was beginning to rise; I was shivering, then sweating, shivering, then sweating. Still, there was nothing to do but drive. So I did.

I decided to take the coastal route instead of going inland, on Highway 17. If I had to spend a few nights on the side of the road, it would be easier near the beaches, the wheat-colored hills. I put on the radio, heard that Santa Cruz had been destroyed, that the ceiling in the San Francisco airport had collapsed and that many people had been killed. Each report about Santa Cruz was worse than the previous one: the university was on fire, the downtown mall had caved in, people were running through the streets looking for their children, their animals. Mayhem.

Scenes from the Jane Alexander movie *Testament* flooded into my mind. She and her family were living an ordinary suburban life when a nuclear bomb exploded. Her husband was on a business trip; they never saw each other again. Her children died slow, agonizing deaths from radiation poisoning. I watched the movie with my friend Ellen in my lacy white bedroom in Santa Cruz. We were eating popcorn when the movie began; by the end we were numb. The thought that our lives could be destroyed in one second, the fact that there were enough nuclear weapons to destroy the world a hundred times over, terrified us. What do we do with this information? we asked each other. How do we brush our teeth, take out the garbage, eat Cheerios, when all of life is hanging on a fragile, quivering thread?

We never answered the questions. The next day I got up, brushed my teeth, took out the garbage, ate cereal for breakfast. I didn't know what to do, so I did nothing. Eventually I buried the fear beneath the composted egg-shells in the garden.

A gas station in Pacifica was open. I filled up my tank, headed for Santa Cruz, listened to the radio, wondered where Matt was. If he was alive. No time was given for the collapse of the ceiling in the airport. Matt's plane arrived nine minutes after the earthquake. Could he have been in the terminal, under the ceiling? I felt as if I were driving in a dream, listening to the radio in a dream. This was not me, my community, my lover, my friends, my life. Everything had been fine when I left Santa Cruz six hours ago. That was my life; this was not.

I turned onto Alice Street, not knowing if I was going to find my house intact or in a blue clapboard rubble.

Intact.

Wind chimes from Big Sur still hanging on the porch. They stood still, innocent, as if nothing had happened since I last saw them.

I opened the door. Jane, my housesitter, was sweeping up the fragments of plates, glasses, vases, burgundy decanters of my great-grandmother's. Blanche was hiding in the closet. I walked into the bathroom and, for the first time since I was twelve, spent the evening draped on the bathroom floor, throwing up.

Matt called at ten o'clock. He was standing in the phone booth at Park 'n Fly at the airport, had been trying to get through to me for hours, uncertain whether I was at the hotel, where they told him I'd checked in, or in Santa Cruz. Call your mother, he said. She's convinced that you were on the bridge. I love you, he said, I'll come right home.

My mother, whom I could not contact because the phone lines were jammed, spent the night with a magnifying glass in front of the television set. She knew I'd driven to San Francisco that day, but did not know that the Bay Bridge was not part of my route. Frightened that I had been on the bridge when it collapsed, she tried to read the license plates of the cars that were hanging from girders, flattened like recycled soup cans on the lower level.

We had seven hundred aftershocks—further earthquakes—in the weeks to come. None of my close friends lost their houses. All of them lost the security that comes from believing that life is predictable, that what you have and who you are today will be what you have and who you are tomorrow. They began to act in ways that I acted as a child, peppering their sentences with "never," "always," and "from now on":

"I'm never driving under a raised freeway."

"From now on, I will know where my son is at every moment of the day."

"I'm never driving to San Francisco again."

"I'm never driving over another bridge as long as I live."

"My relatives from Los Angeles will have to come here because I am never going there."

Matt and I bought portable phones so that we would *never* be out of touch again. I promised myself that I would *always* keep my car filled with gas.

The cleaving earth had turned us into children who could not depend on our families, the ground we walked on, for safety. We were frightened, anxious, irrational. Sleep was impossible. Psychologists call it post-traumatic stress disorder, said it could last six weeks or six months. But it was so familiar to me, this irrationality, this insistent need to protect myself from the possibility of disaster at any moment, that I felt as if I'd been living with post-traumatic stress disorder all my life, and that finally, everyone I knew, met on the street, talked to in a store— the entire community of Santa Cruz—mirrored the child's world I knew.

I was alone during the earthquake. It didn't matter that I was a writer, a teacher, a friend, that my book was about to be published. Nothing could protect me from walking through the Saint Francis in the dark, from spending hours not knowing whether my cat, my friends, my lover, were dead or alive. From the rawness and the vulnerability of knowing in a way I had never known that everything I counted on, everything I loved, could be destroyed in seven seconds. And what would I be left with? The same thing I am always left with:

Body. Feelings. Mind. Soul.

Not things, not titles, not work, not relationships.

The ways I allow myself to experience what is happening. Or the ways I defend myself against it, bury the fear beneath the eggshells in the garden.

My natural inclination is to bury the feelings I would prefer not to feel. After twenty years of therapy, thirteen years of spiritual practice, after knowing that the only way out is through, the movement is still away from what is difficult—even when what is difficult is true, is real—and toward pretending, toward denial. As if burying my feelings will make them go away. As if what is unseen has no consequences.

In the weeks following the earthquake, as I traveled back and forth to Berkeley, it was as if I were suspended between radically different worlds. The earthquake had not affected Berkeley; our friends there were not experiencing a lack of trust in the ground they walked on.

We'd go to a gathering, and terror was absent; people were joking about the earthquake. They felt the false safety that comes from believing that life today will be the same as life tomorrow. Santa Cruz was still heaving with aftershocks. The downtown mall had indeed collapsed; the city was wrecked, in rubble. You couldn't look away, you couldn't pretend that a disaster had not happened. Could not happen again in five years, next week. Any second.

Many people left California after the 1989 earthquake. Still more after the 1993 earthquake. Matt and I talked about it, our friends talked about it. We considered moving to New Mexico, Colorado, Oregon, Australia. The Southwest had nuclear power plants; the Northwest had fog and rain ten months of the year; Australia had holes in the ozone. My mother wanted me to fly to New York, stay with her until the aftershocks stopped. Better yet, she'd say, move back to New York. You have to be crazy to keep living in California. There are only going to be more earthquakes, and next time you really might be on the Bay Bridge. New York, Mom? I'd say. You think I'd be safer in New York City than in Santa Cruz?

We stayed in California because it was home. Because there is no escape from the fact that at any moment, because of any number of things, events, people, your life can change completely. Because there is no such thing as finding safety outside yourself, not even in the earth.

During the Vietnam War I was in love with the vice-president of the university. When we went on strike outside Tressider Student Union, he wore a black armband to show his alliance with the students that had been killed at Kent State University. I wore a black armband, too, but I didn't feel the fire of protest. I wore black earrings to match my armband. The sixties did not turn me into a political activist. They did introduce me to Birkenstocks and tie-dyed skirts, taking psychedelic drugs, growing underarm hair, eating Continental yogurt, and having sex with men who smiled at me over tofu sandwiches in Greenstreet Restaurant. The sixties gave me Ram Dass's books and a nonstop flight from JFK to Bombay.

It was in India, in discovering that the work of living was seeing through the veils between what I identified as me—my personality, my body, my history, my work, my relationships—and what people called God or soul or essence, that the sixties had their most profound effect on me. Before India I didn't believe that there was anything beyond the desire to be thin and beautiful and famous and loved. Should I ever achieve those things, I believed my life would have meaning, that the attempts to achieve them *gave* my life meaning. After India I kept trying to be thin and famous and beautiful, but I knew then, just as I know now, that when I look outside myself for meaning, I get what outside things can give me—a false kind of nourishment. Full and not satisfied. Full and looking for more. So I keep traveling the inner journey, keep searching for what the Sufis call "the pearl beyond price."

People come to me because they believe that being thin will dissolve their pain. The people who fill my workshops have tried everything: diets, fasts, exercise, no-fat regimes, stomach stapling, jaw wiring, anorexia, bulimia, suicide. Most of them have been thin at least once in their lives. But they cannot give up the dream that something they can touch, accomplish, control will fill the hole, feed their hungry hearts.

It is hard—excruciating—to give up the dream, even when it's already come true once, twice, three times and been empty. Every time a dream proves disappointing, we replace it with a bigger dream. Okay, we say, I was thin ten years ago, but I didn't have work that I loved, I didn't have a lover. Now I have those things, and I'm certain that being thin will release me. I'll finally be able to stop thinking about my body and have a life.

When I stand in front of a room filled with people who are counting on being thin to give meaning to their lives and ask, "What brings you peace? What brings you joy?" none of them answer that it is being thin. But knowing that being thin hasn't done it, won't ever do it—that resolving the issues with food won't, in the end, fill the hole—is frightening. And I understand why.

This week I saw a red chenille sweater in a store window in Manhattan. Burnished, soft. Long enough to wear with leggings, trousers, long skirts, jeans. On sale for half its regular price. I was with Matt when I saw it. We were on our way to dinner, and the thought of taking off my coat, sweater, turtleneck, and earrings was burdensome. Besides, Matt is an impatient shopper, and he doesn't think I need any more sweaters. Although I tell him that need is not part of the shopping experience, I know that if I want to receive any pleasure from trying on clothes, it is best to be without my husband. So I held the sweater up to my face, my body, saw that it glowed against my skin, and decided to come back and try it on the next day with my favorite shopping partner, my mother.

Unfortunately, I forgot about it the next day, and by the time it occurred to me the following day, it was too late to get to the store. On the third day we flew out of the city on an early morning flight. (I realize from this description that I do not sound like a serious shopper. Serious shoppers do not forget about thrilling articles of clothing that are half price, can be worn with everything they have, and have the potential to make their lives luscious. But from the moment my mother and I first walked into My Darling Daughter and I tried on a forest green pinafore with sprigs of violets, to the day I walked into Chandler's Shoe Store and bought my first pair of heels for twenty-six dollars, up to and beyond the time I lost my hair and discovered that buying hats with big purple flowers and gold ribbons made me feel vital again, shopping has occupied a place next to food in my life as an activity that promises sensual pleasure, excitement, and relief from whatever is disturbing me.)

So, the sweater is in New York, and I am in Aruba with Matt on his company's retreat. Making long-distance phone calls is expensive (five dollars a minute) and time-consuming (ten minutes to get through to the long-distance operator). I don't have the number of the store, so I would have to pay for the information call as well. I didn't try on the sweater, so I can't be positive that I will like it as well on my body as I did on the shelf. It's probably not on sale anymore. In fact, it's probably not in the store anymore. And Matt is right: I don't need another sweater.

Given that all this is true, why, in ninety-degree, humid weather, as I gaze at the turquoise Caribbean Sea, am I thinking about a red chenille sweater?

I ask people in workshops what they would be thinking about if they were not thinking about food and their bodies ninety percent of the time. What they would be doing with their days, their evenings, if they weren't planning, dreaming, dieting, bingeing?

Most of them say their lives would be fabulous. They say they could walk down a street, swing their thin hips, and feel confident. They say they could wake up in the morning liking themselves, could go to sleep with their spouses unashamed of their bodies. They say they could finally focus on other things.

What other things? I ask.

Relationships. Work. Living space. Quality of life.

More goals, more dreams. Different than being thin. And exactly the same. More ways to keep the restlessness occupied.

The desire, the need, for something to fill the hole is so intense that we can't allow ourselves to feel the emptiness of knowing that nothing we want, nothing we reach for, will do it.

I dreamed of being thin and I lost weight. I dreamed of being a writer and became one. I dreamed of reaching hundreds of thousands of people and was given that opportunity. I dreamed of being in a relationship with someone I loved, and now I am. Each one of those dreams fueled my energy, focused my passion—and proved ultimately disappointing. Not for what they are—body, work, love—but for what I wanted them to be: the end of my search, the meaning of my life, the basis of self-value.

Goals and dreams are important, necessary; they provide movement, inspiration. But if achieving them was truly what we were hungering for, it would be enough to be thin once. To have one beautiful sweater. We keep getting what we want and wanting more, and although wanting what we don't have is a condition of mind, it is also an indication that we are wanting something that cannot be touched, controlled, accomplished, in the usual ways.

If I wasn't thinking of red chenille, what would I be thinking about? What would I be feeling? I might be in touch with the longing to be home instead of in Aruba. I might remember the day in July when my mother-in-law asked me if I was going with Matt on this trip and I said no. She told me a story about a couple that got divorced because the wife didn't participate in her husband's life. I might remember the cloud of fear as I sat there, eating spinach pasta with wild mushrooms, listening to her story.

Might remember the plastic shrunken head I hung in my bedroom when I was eight. I told my father that it represented his mother, my grandmother, thinking that I was being cute, mimicking my mother, who wouldn't accompany us to my grandmother's, who wouldn't participate in my father's life.

I might remember and feel the pain, the hopelessness of watching my parents grow increasingly violent with each other. Might remember that I blamed it on my mother, believed that if she could be conciliatory, would accompany us when we went to the Airline Diner for breakfast or to the Bronx on Sunday afternoons, we could be a family, they could stay together.

I might have a visual image of hard-edged metal and sandpaper; might feel the sensations of sandpaper—the grinding, the blasting, the intense effort to take away the edges. How hard I try to keep myself in line, to smooth the ways I stick out, to run over anything that makes me different, that causes others discomfort. The fear that if I allow myself to feel what I feel, to know what I know, I will lose everything, everyone.

If I wasn't thinking of red chenille, I might be aware of my desire to have the marriage my parents didn't, no matter what the cost. Might allow myself to feel the intensity with which I push away everything I don't want to feel. Fear. Hopelessness. I might remember being a child who loved her mother with a feeling so big that it was like exploding comets and galaxies and the color of peaches. I might remember when I learned that I couldn't, shouldn't, was absolutely not allowed to be that big, that my love had to be contained and shaped and determined by what the other wanted.

I might remember my father, how I depended on him for laughter and affection, for joy and a safe place. How he played monster from the green sea with me, and how attuned I became to what he needed from me, who I needed to be so that he would keep loving me. I might remember our implicit agreement—he could be smart and powerful, while I played the girly dependent. I would stay small so that he could stay big. I would stay empty so that he could fill me. In return I received nothing less than my life. As I grew older, and we stopped playing monster from the green sea, and we stopped reading *The Little Engine That Could*, our relationship was sustained, in part, by a different kind of wanting: the wanting of things. Patti Playpals. Rabbit fur jackets. Purple angora sweaters.

A red chenille sweater. Wanting things that could easily be given, be gotten, rather than wanting what I knew I couldn't have from either of my parents: being seen, being met. Being valued for the fullness I already embodied.

As I sit at the table in our hotel room, I might notice the terror that arises as soon as I start feeling full, big, powerful. I'll lose my daddy's love. Matt's love. I might notice then what fear actually feels like. Brown ropy cords wrapped around my chest, squeezing my heart, my muscles. I might allow myself to breathe into the fear instead of push it away. Might notice that when I feel the constriction, it changes, opens into a kind of dark fluid tunnel in which I am sliding. And if I allow myself to breathe, to slide, to keep sliding, if I don't get frightened by unexpected sensations, I might notice that I land in a meadow where it is night and the sky is an explosion of comets, whole galaxies. And that the explosions, the light, are not only outside me, but inside as well. If I didn't at that point think I had gone completely mad, if I didn't try to pull myself back into my everyday world of fear and tightness, if I kept allowing the unfolding, I might breathe into the galaxy of my body and feel endless as space, deep as indigo.

In Room 418 of the Sonesta Hotel, I might remember, if only for a second, who I am when I am not afraid of knowing what I know and feeling what I feel. I might feel such value in that moment that I would trust that no one could take it away from me because no one gave it to me to begin with.

If I wasn't thinking of red chenille.

If I didn't believe that being thin could save me.

But I do. We do. We live in a culture that completely supports our desires, the things we believe will give us value. Being thin. Being loved. Dressing in red chenille.

Anne Wilson Schaef: "The society in which we live needs addictions, and its very essence fosters addictions. It fosters addictions because the best-adjusted person in the society is the person who is not dead and not alive, just numb, a zombie. When you are dead, you are not able to do the work of the society. When you are fully alive, you are constantly saying no to many of the processes of the society: the racism, the polluted environment, the nuclear threat, the arms race, drinking unsafe water, eating carcinogenic food."

The work is to allow yourself to know what you know, to be who you are when you are not defining yourself by the size of your body and the content of your fears and whether you are loved on a particular day.

The work is to allow yourself not to know. To understand that you believe that being thin, being loved, is going to make you happy because you have replaced something you can get (being thin) with something you don't know if you can get (the absolute knowledge that you deserve to exist). You have been told that being thin will save you, and it is lonely and frightening to question the beliefs of the majority.

The work is to honestly inquire into the nature of your experience. What is it that brings you peace, joy, value? Is it money, is it being thin, is it a red chenille sweater? The work is not to judge those things. Or to not have those things. They are fine for what they are; they provide what things outside you can provide. But if you have been thin once and have gained weight and everything in your life, your heart, and your energy, all your time, all your dreams, are pointing toward, waiting for the moment, when you are thin again, you are caught in a cycle of false hopes, beliefs, illusions. You are living in the world of lies. Because when you think that being thin or being, having, doing any one thing is going to fill the emptiness, you are not allowing for the possibility that you are as big as a galaxy, as ripe as a peach, as endless as space. You are not allowing for the possibility—the reality—that you are already full. That fullness, joy, value, peace does not depend on a body size or a bank account or the whims of another person. On anything but your own ability to recognize and honor them in yourself as they already exist.

You begin from where you are: You want to be thin; you want a red sweater; you want more money; you want a soul mate. Then you travel: You ask; you explore; you dive.

We keep looking for a safe place. For most women it is the fantasy of life as a thin person. For women who are or who have already been thin, the illusion gets projected onto careers, children, lovers, clothes, success, money. The ultimate illusion, of course, is when all else fails, the earth is safe. We can count on the sun and the wind, on spring following winter, on red-winged blackbirds slicing through the sky. But that, too, is a lie.

Two months before the Santa Cruz earthquake, Matt and I bought a house in Berkeley. An enchanted house with three fireplaces and a crooked, mosaic bathroom floor. Our move-in date was the day after Christmas, December 26, 1989. The first time we walked into the house after the earthquake, I became hysterical. If there is an earthquake, I said, there is no way out of the house. The fireplaces will topple on each doorway, the decks will collapse, we'll be trapped. I want to move, I told Matt. It's not safe here.

He answered that if I still felt that way in six months, we would sell the house and move. Then he asked me where I would like to go.

We went through the litany of cities, countries. We talked about moving back to Santa Cruz, since according to the seismologists, the Big One had already happened there, and it would be another hundred years before another Big One. Berkeley and the entire San Francisco Bay area were, however, long overdue. According to the latest reports, there was a sixty percent chance that an earthquake of seven or greater on the Richter scale would level the Bay area in the next thirty years. We consulted maps and discovered that our enchanted house sat directly on the Hayward Fault.

I was a wild woman. Raw, fragile, jumpy. Every time I drove over the Bay Bridge, I called my mother on the car phone, convinced that God would not let me die if I was talking to my mother. I glued vases, decanters, perfume bottles to shelves; I nailed bookcases, armoires to walls; I placed water, flashlights, transistor radios, cash, at different places in the house. Kept a pair of shoes and a crowbar underneath my bed in case we needed to wedge our way out of the wreckage of glass, bricks, books. I prepared myself. And then I lived in fear.

A few months ago, I woke up one morning to a blazing orange glow outside our window. Curious but not frightened, I yawned, stretched, padded over to the window, opened the curtains. Saw the house next door to us, two feet away, burning down. The screened-in porch collapsed as I watched. I screamed for Matt to wake up, get his clothes on. Call 911, get Blanche, leave the house. I knew that the fire could reach our house within five minutes and that we had less than that to gather whatever we could and get out. Matt grabbed his portable computer, put Blanche in the cat carrier, took his wedding ring, and walked to the front door. I tore through the house gathering thirty years of journals, most of which were 8½ by 11 heavy, cumbersome books. I ran with them up the stairs. Grabbed the computer disks of my current book. As I passed the living room, I remembered my great-grandmother's silver overlay bottles, my grandmother's earrings, our wedding album. My childhood pictures, letters from adolescence, the black enamel music box my father gave me when I was six. The vase from Russia, my mother's cameo, my wedding rings. My computer. The stuffed pencil Peg left me when she died. I kept running to the window to see if the fire department had come, if the fire had reached the sidewalk between our houses. Kept tearing up and down the stairs with photographs, jewelry, journals. Remembered my childhood stuffed animals—a squirrel with a nut between his paws—and ran downstairs again. Found the squirrel, and the pink bassett hound with the button eyes falling off. Decided to take the black corduroy skating outfit I had when I was ten. Saw the neon light Matt had given me for our first Valentine's Day together, with GR & MW inscribed in the middle of a heart. Took that as well. Then I remembered my wedding dress in the basement. Ran down to find it, saw my childhood rocking chair. The tutu I wore in the ballet recital when I was six. Carried all three of them up the stairs. Breathless and exhausted from so many trips up and down the stairs in five minutes, I decided to leave everything in the house and go outside, where Matt was standing with the neighbors.

The fire was out; the back half of a neighbor's house was in craggy, charred pieces on the ground. Through the open front door I could see a pink paisley wing chair lying on its side, half the cushion burned. They told us that one of their sons put his cigarette out on the porch, but it smoldered and eventually set the porch on fire.

A cigarette. I'd been bracing myself for an earthquake, not a fire. I'd spent five years believing that if my house was destroyed, it would be because the earth cleaved, not because a seventeen-year-old was careless about a cigarette.

During the California mud slides of 1982, when houses were slipping off their foundations and falling down the hills, a woman Sally knew—Betsy Rollins—decided to move from where she was spending the night, on Cathedral Drive in Aptos, to a higher, safer place, in Ben Lomond, fifteen miles away. She drove in the sleeting rain, seeking safety. She arrived in the house at ten p.m. At eleven-thirty, the house in which she was sleeping slid off its foundation and collapsed. She died instantly. On Cathedral Drive, in Aptos, the house she evacuated stood strong, steady.

I sat on the sidewalk, with my peach sweatpants under my flannel nightgown, under my lime green sweater, and I considered the facts. I thought about Betsy Rollins. About calling my mother every time I drove over the bridge. The thud in my chest at the slightest tremor in the house. The fear of the earth being destroyed and life as we know it ending. The firemen walked past me; my neighbors returned to their houses. Matt brought Blanche inside the house. He made a phone call. He came back outside. I was still sitting on the sidewalk. He eyed me with concern. Is it stress, honey? he asked. I shook my head.

I was beginning to understand that even if I had managed to remove my journals, vases, rings, photographs, bottles, cameo, music box, rocking chair, neon light, wedding dress, skating dress, tutu, and stuffed animals from the house, I couldn't have saved them—our street is too narrow for fire trucks and cars. We would have been forced to flee on foot with Blanche, computer disks, computer, wedding rings (perhaps the cameo, a journal, a pile of photographs), and our lives. And I also realized that anything that could be eaten by flames in a matter of minutes wasn't mine. Now or ever. Including Matt and Blanche. Life itself was a huge, temporary gift, and if I lived in fear that the whole thing could be taken away, and if I actually had the audacity to believe that I knew how it was going to happen, then I was living a lie. I was living in a world constructed by my fantasies, my fears. I could spend my life preparing and living in perpetual dread of the worst imaginable nightmare, and in five minutes something I never anticipated could grab me by the feet, the hair, the heart, and knock me over.

The thought—no, the truth—that my life depended on whether some kid I didn't know put out his cigarette made the choices extraordinarily clear: Surrender to the apparent randomness of life. Accept the interdependence of my life on other lives. Continue to act on those issues about which I feel passionate. *Or* take all precautions against a disaster that may never happen until I am rocked with an event for which there is no preparation. Do everything I can to fit myself into the needs of people I love, and evoke anger, pain, envy, anyway. Try to protect myself from being hurt and get hurt nonetheless. Construct a world based on fear and fantasy and the illusion of a safe place and discover, again and again, that there is no safe place.

Live my life as only I can live it or live a lie.

Martha Graham: "There is a vitality, a life force, an energy, a quickening that is translated through you into action. And because there is only one of you in all time, this expression is unique. And if you block it, it will never exist through any other medium, and be lost. The world will not have it. It is not your business to determine how good it is, or how valuable, or how it compares with other expressions. It is your business to keep the channel open. You have to keep open and aware directly to the urges that actuate you. Keep the channel open."

We close the channel by believing that we can control and prepare for the future. We close it when we don't act on our passions. We close it by being afraid. We close it by thinking that if we allow ourselves to open it, no one will love us—we will be too full, too powerful, too radiant. We close it by believing that peace and joy and truth and value are not our birthright. We close it by compulsive eating, compulsive shopping, compulsive anything. The purpose of compulsion, in fact, was to close the channel at a time in our lives when it was not safe to keep it open.

Despite my valiant efforts to the contrary, I know that the purpose of life is not to be safe. It is to be open. To be dedicated to the truth, to the joy as it streams through your life. Because if you are not, then no matter what you have, you will always want more, you will be forever hungry. And if you are, then no matter what happens, you will one day discover that you are who you have been hungering for. It has been you, not the food you eat, the clothes you buy, the people you love, the money you make. For lifetimes, for eons, for as long as it takes for a mountain to become a mountain, it has always been you.

You are the feast.

You.

Epilogue:
Seven Remembrances

Five years ago, I was teaching at Omega Institute for the weekend, and one of the workshop attendees was camping out. On our second day together, she told the group that she had never cared about the earth. She littered the ground, didn't recycle newspaper or glass, and threw waste in the river. But during the night, something had changed. The words people had spoken the day before sifted into her consciousness, and she awoke with a trace of self-kindness. "Perhaps I don't deserve to treat myself so badly," she said. She mentioned that she felt a new tenderness for herself, and that she didn't know why or how, but it translated to the earth; she'd picked up a discarded Coke can on the way to the meeting. "I know that may not sound like a big thing to most of you, but for me, it marks a change because I *wanted* to pick up the can. I didn't do it because it was the right thing to do—I did it because something opened inside me. I'm usually too busy feeling that I'm not getting enough of what I want or need to give a damn about what's happening around me."

I am not an expert on treating the earth or myself with tenderness. Sometimes, when I gain five pounds, I act as if I've committed a felony, and when I read the newspaper, I often feel paralyzed by the judgment that I am spending my time on the inner journey when, in a matter of years, there may be no planet left to journey *on*. But I try to remember this woman's glistening face when I question the connection between the inner and outer life, or feel hopeless about change of any kind.

I also try to remember the following:

The sweetest gift, the only gift, we can give ourselves, our communities, the earth is our fullest, truest presence. Simply put, our presence is who we are, or would be, if we weren't always trying to be someone else.

The process is the goal. If we do what we do because it is politically correct or nice or will someday make us happy, someday will never come, and we will have wasted our lives waiting.

Longing is the soul's way of saying "I know you thought this was it, but it's not. Don't stop here." Longing is the voice of the universe (i.e., what many people call God) desiring to manifest its fullness through us; it is not an expression of the wanting mind gone wild.

We do not have to give up thinness or success or

love when we admit these things don't do what we thought they would. Telling the truth makes it possible to fully (and for the first time) enjoy those things because we begin to understand that our lives do not depend on them, which makes us less frightened of losing them.

When I am not hanging on to love or success, I actually have moments of being deliriously happy. So will you.

We can't understand or move through what we refuse to examine. It's not until we admit we are lost that there is even a possibility of discovering a new way.

We already have true nourishment; *we* are the nourishment we have been searching for.

We think we know what will make us happy, but we are usually wrong. We think joy comes by acquiring things or relationships or love, but it doesn't. (If it did, we would already be happy.) Joy comes when we remember the qualities from which we cut ourselves off long ago. Value, strength, will, compassion, love. Socrates called them the eternal verities; he said you cannot teach people to have courage or love or strength, but that we know these things by remembering them.

It makes me feel good to think of Socrates walking around the city of Athens teaching people that true nourishment comes by remembering who they are, not from getting new white togas and shiny gold belts.

Finally, we are not helping anyone when we pretend to feel less, have less, or be less than we are.

The world will not fall apart if we let ourselves express our vastness. It is more likely the world will stop falling apart when we do.

Acknowledgments

My editor, Carole DeSanti, held the vision of this book through my illness and darkest times. For her persistence, her brilliance, and her belief in me, I am grateful beyond words and roses. My jewel of an agent, Angela Miller, became a trusted friend and a wise reader during the writing of this book, and it is my great good fortune to know her.

As always, it is my friends who sustain me when I need a look, a word, a presence to remind me that there is life beyond this chapter or this feeling. I would like to thank: Sara Friedlander for her willingness to let the story be told, and for her undying love; Jace Schinderman, my first real friend, for being there always; Joanna Macy for seeing and believing in me when I most needed to be seen and believed in; Natalie Goldberg, Meredith Maran, and Katy Hutchins for a first read-through of the book; Prem Siri Khalsa for being my girliest of friends;

Acknowledgments

Sil Reynolds and Francie White for being my wise co-horts; and Lew Fein for everything, always.

This book would be a completely different book were it not for Hameed Ali and the Diamond Heart School in Berkeley. I owe many of the concepts expressed herein to the Diamond Approach. My life has flowered and become mine since I discovered it, and my joy feels as big as a universe of falling stars. For opening the door of this universe and for being her own bright light, I am forever grateful to Taj Glantz. I would also like to thank the members of my small group for consistency and support, and for providing a place where truth is always honored, indeed expected. And then there is Jeanne Hay, who manages to embody whatever quality I need in the moment. For holding the journey with such love, and for being herself like the fragrance of plumeria flowers, I feel gratitude beyond measure.

Others to whom I am grateful are: Terry Kupers for his integrity and belief in having an embarrassment of riches; Karin Lippert for launching my work and for being on my side when no one else was; Elaine Koster, my publisher, and Lisa Johnson, the publicity director, at Dutton for their constant support; M. A. Bjarkman, Rae Baskin and The Conference Works, and Cindy Lambert of The Family Institute of Maine for producing the Breaking Free workshops, and for growing with me through the years; and Lynne August for saving my life.

The courage of the women who share their lives with me, both at the workshops and in letters, gives me inspiration, hope, and joy, and I feel a never-ending gratitude and respect for them. Karen Russell, the woman who came to a workshop and subsequently lost three hundred pounds, gave thousands of women the concrete proof that reclaiming their lives was possible. I will never forget her.

I can't imagine my life without Maureen Nemeth, my trusted office manager, friend, locator of potato sacks and everything else I need. I am thankful daily for her feisty humor, her loyalty, her intelligence, and her deep love of the work we do.

And last as well as first, Matt Weinstein listened to every word of this book at least three times. For never ceasing to believe in it or me, for loving me truly through sickness and health, and for being like the color of an island sunrise in mid-September, I feel a thousand times blessed.

For information on the lectures and workshops offered by Geneen Roth and her colleagues at Breaking Free®, or to receive a list of audio- and videotapes, please contact:

Breaking Free
P.O. Box 2852
Santa Cruz, California 95063

(408) 685-8601; fax (408) 685-8602

**Visit the author at
www.GeneenRoth.com**

*Breaking Free is a registered trademark® of Geneen Roth